HEALTH CARE IN A CONTEXT OF CIVIL RIGHTS

INSTITUTE OF MEDICINE

NATIONAL ACADEMY PRESS
Washington, D.C. 1981

NOTICE The project that is the subject of this report was approved by the Governing Board of the National Research Council, whose members are drawn from the Councils of the National Academy of Sciences, the National Academy of Engineering, and the Institute of Medicine. The members of the committee responsible for the report were chosen for their special competences and with regard for appropriate balance.

This report has been reviewed by a group other than the authors according to procedures approved by a Report Review Committee consisting of members of the National Academy of Sciences, the National Academy of Engineering, and the Institute of Medicine.

Supported by the Department of Health and Human Services Contract No. 282-78-0163-EJM, T.O. 14.

Publication IOM 81-04

The Institute of Medicine was chartered in 1970 by the National Academy of Sciences to enlist distinguished members of the appropriate professions in the examination of policy matters pertaining to the health of the public. In this, the Institute acts under both the Academy's 1863 congressional charter responsibility to be an adviser to the federal government and its own initiative in identifying issues of medical care, research, and education.

Library of Congress Catalog Card Number 81-84682

International Standard Book Number 0-309-03195-8

Available from

NATIONAL ACADEMY PRESS
2101 Constitution Avenue, N.W.
Washington D.C. 20418

Printed in the United States of America

COMMITTEE FOR A STUDY OF THE HEALTH CARE OF RACIAL/ETHNIC MINORITIES AND HANDICAPPED PERSONS

Chairman

Rosemary A. STEVENS, Ph.D., Professor of History and Sociology of Science, University of Pennsylvania, Philadelphia

Members

Rodolfo ALVAREZ, Ph.D., Professor of Sociology, University of California at Los Angeles

Susan M. DANIELS, Ph.D., Head, Department of Rehabilitation Counseling, Louisiana State University Medical Center, New Orleans

Linda K. DEMLO, Ph.D., Administrative Scholar, Veterans Administration, Washington, D.C.

Jonathan E. FIELDING, M.D., M.P.H., Professor of Pediatrics and Public Health, Center for Health Enhancement Education and Research, Center for the Health Sciences, University of California at Los Angeles

John W. HATCH, Dr.P.H., Associate Professor, School of Public Health, University of North Carolina, Chapel Hill

Frank P. HOCHMAN, M.D., Medical Practitioner, Fremont, California

Sylvia LAW, J.D., Professor of Law, New York University Law School, New York

David MECHANIC, Ph.D., Acting Dean, Faculty of Arts and Sciences, Rutgers University, New Brunswick, New Jersey

Howard NEWMAN, J.D., Member in Residence, Institute of Medicine, National Academy of Sciences (Mr. Newman was not an active committee member after June 1980.)

Helen RODRIGUEZ-TRIAS, M.D., Director, Children and Youth Comprehensive Medical Care Program, Roosevelt Hospital, New York

Gerald D. ROSENTHAL, Ph.D., Director, National Center for Health Services Research, Department of Health and Human Services, Hyattsville, Maryland

William A. SPENCER, M.D., President, Texas Institute for Rehabilitation, Texas Medical Center, Houston

Leonard I. STEIN, M.D., Professor of Psychiatry, University of
Wisconsin, Madison

Charles WATTS, M.D., Assistant Director, Lincoln Community Health
Center, Durham, North Carolina

Study Staff

Bradford H. Gray, Ph.D., Study Director, Senior Professional Associate
Jana H. Surdi, Professional Associate
Paul M. Campbell, Professional Associate
Kathryn G. King, Research Associate
Bob McConnaughey, Student Intern
Kenneth Wing, J.D., Special Consultant

CONTENTS

PREFACE

This report is peculiarly American. The committee was brought together at the request at the Office for Civil Rights, Department of Health and Human Services, to review information about observable disparities or inequalities in health care affecting two large, dissimilar, and distinctive groups--members of social/ethnic minorities and handicapped persons--whose only link is through civil rights legislation. Minority groups are a primary target of legislation under Title VI of the Civil Rights Act; handicapped individuals under Section 504 of the Rehabilitation Act. We were asked not to draw conclusions as to whether and in what respects members of these groups were subject to racial discrimination or discrimination by virtue of handicapping condition. Nevertheless, the choice of these two groups--whose conjunction would make little sense in considering policies in any other country's health care system--was clearly generated by interests as to whether and in what respects civil rights procedures ought to be extended in the health care system.

As a committee we have tried to be objective in the collection, analysis, and presentation of our data. Yet the subject matter of this report is value-laden. The ambiguities, complexities, and tensions in American health care make discussions of equality particularly difficult. Who is to say what is fair or unfair in the receipt of health services in the United States, and on what basis? There is no consensus, at least as yet. What disparities in the receipt of care are to be regarded as just or unjust? What differences are to be legally prohibited under civil rights legislation? Nearly all Americans would claim that at least some health services should be available to all members of the population or even perhaps that, as far as possible, health services should be distributed "equitably." But how does one approach questions of equity? Does equity mean equal numbers of visits for all groups? Equal length of life? Because the structure of the American health care system is not designed to deliver services equally to all members of the population, it makes little sense to assume that, with a little tinkering, it would.

Moreover, health is not the same as the receipt of medical care. Factors extraneous to the health care system, such as income, diet, smoking, genetic heritage, and stress, may powerfully affect an individual's condition. Even in countries where equality of services is a goal, as in Britain, there remain striking differences in the health of different groups.* Britain's analysis of health by social (occupational) class raises yet another set of uncertainties. Discussion of social class differences is faintly un-American; race and handicapping conditions provide more urgent classifications, as reflected in civil rights concerns. Even the choice of groups for study (and available data) reflects cultural beliefs.

Yet it is precisely <u>because</u> the questions are difficult and value-laden, and because of the empirical complexities of investigation, that this report has been undertaken. If serious discussion about equalities and inequalities in American health care is to take place, review of available evidence about disparities in American medical care is obviously essential. Members of this committee agreed to give their time to this study because of concern about the adequacy of care to various members of the population, signified here as care to minorities and handicapped individuals. Equity is an important value in the society in which we live. Access to health care ought to be assured to all members of the population. This study reveals serious imbalances in care received by different groups. As financial resources for medical care become more limited, particularly in programs such as Medicaid that disproportionately affect needy individuals, it becomes correspondingly more important to articulate the social goals of health care programs and to measure their effects on different populations. By arraying available evidence about disparities in health and health care--scanty though this evidence often is--this report is a beginning of a process of discussion and debate (and better data collection) out of which health and civil rights policies can be more openly addressed.

Civil rights approaches also need considerable discussion and clarification as they apply to health care issues. We do not mean to imply in this report that disparities in care in and of themselves are civil rights issues in the legal sense. If the law's objective is to eliminate purposeful discrimination on the basis of race or physical handicap in the delivery of health care, then it will not suffice simply to discover or show that there are significant disparities in the use of, or access to, health care. As one of our legal critics pointed out, many observers believe that the major civil rights problem today is not conscious and overt discrimination, but rather the more subtle problem associated with a pattern of racially neutral decisions that have racially disparate consequences. The problem here may be a structural one of institutional indifference or insensitivity to the concerns of racial or ethnic minorities or other constituencies not represented in the decision-making process. From this standpoint, perhaps the most effective regulatory action would be to require the decision makers, in various health planning contexts at least, to

---

*<u>Inequalities in Health</u>, Report of a Research Working Group (Sir Douglas Black, chairman), (London: Department of Health and Social Security, August 1980).

assess the likely consequences of proposed actions on access to and utilization of health care services by racial and ethnic minorities or other disparate groups.

This and similar points of debate can only be reached persuasively, however, after careful review of available evidence. We show here the evidence on disparities that now exists and note the serious short- comings (sometimes conflicts) in this evidence. Adequate data are prerequisites to civil rights enforcement activities under present legal obligations and to the continuing process of definition of disparities that are to be regarded as unreasonable or illegitimate in terms of civil rights legislation. We need better data in order to think more clearly about civil rights and health policy development.

Yet it would be a paltry excuse to use the absence of good data to avoid raising policy issues at all. What we have done here is to identify (1) areas in which disparities appear to exist in the health care of members of ethnic/minority groups and handicapped populations compared with the general population and (2) areas in which better information is particularly needed. For analytical purposes we have assumed that any evidence of disparity deserves investigation as a potential health policy or civil rights issue.

Given the committee's mandate and time constraints, the report is inevitably "unfinished." Reviewers consulted by the Institute of Medicine and by the committee have chided us, inter alia, for failing to specify empirical questions or conceptual frameworks; for being insufficiently critical of the complexities in health care (and in American society in general) that may well lead to disparities in care; for failing to disentangle the effects of socioeconomic status; for not providing adequate definitions of "ethnicity"; for lack of discussion on the ethical implications of disparities in care; and for suggesting that disparities may imply discrimination.

Some of these criticisms arise from serious inadequacies in the basic data. For example, ethnicity (or handicap), health care, location, and social class are mutually dependent variables, all of which need to be understood in assessing how real and how general differences in health care actually are. Middle-class blacks may have better health care than lower-class non-blacks; poor people may feel discriminated against whether or not they are from a minority group; persons with hearing problems may report different health care experiences in different cities. Unfortunately, as this report shows, most existing studies do not array data (or do not collect data) by all these variables. We need studies of what different subgroups think about health and illness, whom they go to for care, and with what satisfaction and apparent results. Useful classifications of handicapping conditions are only beginning. In many ways the inadequacies in the data reflect a general unwillingness to think about the policy issues. This report is designed to stimulate action on both the policy and the informational fronts.

Some of the criticisms stem from the committee's mandate. We have not developed empirical questions or conceptual frameworks. We have presented an overview of current research findings and survey data on which others may base further investigations. We have assumed that disparities are "problems" in American health care, whether or not these disparities might prove to be quite reasonable in the light of further empirical investigation or interpretations. Some of the criticisms stem from the committee's biases and perceptions in areas where there are differences of opinion. Some errors of presentation or judgment undoubtedly remain. In our thanking a particularly helpful (if feisty) panel of reviewers, it should be observed that it is precisely this continuing process of clarification, dissent, and discussion that this report is designed to provoke.

It is the chairman's prerogative and pleasure to thank all those who have contributed. A study such as this can be an exciting educational as well as working experience; I should like to thank a superb committee.

The bulk of the work rests, however, on staff. We are extremely fortunate in having Bradford H. Gray as study director. Dr. Gray's expertise and experience as a sociologist who has written extensively on ethical issues in health served us well in developing an agenda. He brought focus and discipline to the work of a group that had far more ideas than time or the means to investigate them. He has the appreciation and thanks of the entire committee.

Dr. Gray gives specific thanks below to other important contributors. Here let me just say, thank you, to all of you.

ROSEMARY STEVENS
<u>Chairman</u>

ACKNOWLEDGMENTS

I would like to gratefully acknowledge the contributions of the many people and organizations who provided assistance to this study. As members of the study staff, Jana Surdi drafted materials that eventually became Chapter 4, and Paul Campbell prepared the summary on racial trends in Medicare and Medicaid that is included as Appendix A. As a summer intern, Bob McConnaughey drafted materials on spatial and geographical aspects of the care of minority groups. Professor Kenneth Wing was a consultant to the committee throughout its existence. In addition to his counsel, he prepared two background papers. One is included as Appendix E, while much of the other found its way into Chapter 5. However, he should not be held responsible for the appearance of the final form of the material he provided nor for the departures from strict legal style in the footnotes.

Many people met with the study committee and shared their expertise about various aspects of the study. These include Dr. Lu Ann Aday from the University of Chicago, Dr. Jacob J. Feldman from the National Center for Health Statistics, Dr. Judith Kaspar from the National Center for Health Services Research, Drs. William Scanlon and Jack Hadley from the Urban Institute, and Dr. Donald Muse from the Health Care Financing Administration. At its briefing in Los Angeles, committee members met with Ms. Sylvia Drew Ivie, then of the National Health Law Program; Ms. Marilyn Holle from the Western Center for Law and the Handicapped; Ms. Mary Ashley from the Martin Luther King, Jr. Hospital; Drs. Rosalyn Murov and Steve Tarzynski from the Los Angeles County Hospital; Mr. Stanton Price, Esq.; Mr. Hal Freeman from the DHHS Office for Civil Rights in San Francisco; Ms. Barbara Guajaca from La Clinica Libre; Ms. Ruth Chaidez from Orange County Hospital; Mr. Miguel Lucero of the Chicano Health Institute of Students, Professors and Alumni in Berkeley; Dr. Adrian Ortega from the Edward R. Roybal Comprehensive Health Center; and Ms. Carmen Estrada, Esq., from the Mexican-American Legal Defense and Education Fund.

Many people kindly shared unpublished data, studies, and papers with us. The National Center for Health Statistics was particularly helpful in this regard, as was the staff of the National Health Law Program who generously shared not only their time but also a wide variety of materials--reports, briefs, and correspondence--that they had accumulated in the course of their work. We are grateful to all of the people who shared their experience and research with the committee. This report is much the richer for it. We particularly appreciate the efforts of the people, listed in Appendix F of this report, who prepared testimony for the committee's public meeting.

In addition to the official IOM/NAS review, a number of people contributed to the report by reviewing and commenting on drafts of parts or all of the report. In this regard I am grateful for the assistance of Dr. Ethel Shanas, Dr. T. Franklin Williams, Mr. Peter Hutt, Mr. Peter Labassi, Dr. Peter Budetti, Ms. Helen Darling, Dr. Gretchen Schafft (who also generously shared her experience and knowledge of the literature on blacks and nursing homes), and Professor Richard J. Bonnie.

The support and assistance of our project officer, Dr. John Halverson, and his colleagues at the Office for Civil Rights also is gratefully acknowledged.

Dr. Carleton Evans, Director of the Division of Health Care Services at the Institute of Medicine, made invaluable contributions to the study both through his intellect and by providing a supportive environment in which the staff could work. Ms. Jessica Townsend and Ms. Marie Kerr provided skilled research and editorial assistance at a crucial time in the production of the final manuscript. Ms. Pat Cornwell served the study well in a secretarial capacity through most of its existence. Ms. Naomi Hudson was responsible for the preparation of the final manuscript.

This study was a great challenge for everyone who worked on it. Without the good will and assistance of many people, it could not have been completed. I want to particularly thank Dr. Rosemary Stevens for her tireless, intellectually rigorous, and always cheerful leadership of the committee and support of the staff. We shall both know better next time.

BRADFORD H. GRAY, Ph.D.
Study Director

Chapter 1

INTRODUCTION AND SUMMARY OF CONCLUSIONS

It is well known that Title VI of the Civil Rights Act of 1964 prohibits discrimination on the ground of race, color, or national origin in any program or activity receiving federal financial assistance; Section 504 of the Rehabilitation Act of 1973 similarly prohibits discrimination by reason of handicap. But relatively little is known about the applicability of these laws in federal health care programs. Through most of its existence in the former Department of Health, Education, and Welfare, the Office for Civil Rights (OCR) devoted most of its resources to the field of education. With the creation of the Department of Education, the Office for Civil Rights in the new Department of Health and Human Services (DHHS) appears likely to increase its attention to health care.

Even before the passage of legislation to divide the Department of Health, Education, and Welfare, OCR had a growing concern with issues that arise in health care. It was, for example, involved in major litigation over patterns of racial segregation in the hospitals of New Orleans and was investigating individual health-related complaints as they arose. However, OCR's few excursions into health had not been based on any systematic assessment of where and in what forms serious problems exist, what evidence might be relevant to the topic, and what sources of information are available. OCR asked the Institute of Medicine to appoint a committee to prepare a report on disparities in health services for racial and ethnic minorities and handicapped people. The committee was also requested to indicate additional work needed to further specify problem areas and suggest possible approaches to remedies. This report is the result of the committee's examination of these issues.

The application of civil rights principles to the delivery of health services is taking place in the context of a changing environment of law as well as health care. In only a few decades, the United States has evolved from a society in which racial discrimination was tolerated and even mandated by legal institutions, to one in which the law forbids many forms of discrimination. Private and public institutions are now explicitly encouraged, and in many cases required, to engage in a variety of activities to eliminate discrimination and alleviate effects of past discrimination.

At the same time, the 1960s and 1970s brought rapid changes in the delivery of health care, marked by increased governmental involvement in its provision, financing, and regulation. Although a full commitment to equality has never characterized American health policy, many governmental programs, as well as civil rights laws, are grounded in concerns about inequity. However, serious questions arise whether the present, partial commitments to equality in health care will be maintained in the face of growing concerns about health care costs. The growing preoccupation with cost control creates pressures for changes that may reduce the availability of health care for the groups for whom civil rights protections are most critical.

The transition from recognition of certain rights in principle to their realization in fact and the translation of broad policy mandates into directives for day-to-day decisions about discrimination have provided severe tests for our legal institutions. There are few settled legal principles on which judgments can rest about particular programs, such as those that finance certain health services. Many aspects of civil rights law, even those as fundamental as the scope and applicability of various non-discrimination prohibitions, remain to be settled.

The civil rights debates of the 1960s and 1970s about such concepts as equal access, equal opportunity, or equality of results in areas of education, employment, housing, and voting rights are likely to be replayed if more active civil rights enforcement develops in health. Yet, it is not clear under what circumstances factual disparities in the provision of care by hospitals and other providers will be considered by the courts to be a result of unlawful discrimination and, if discrimination is identified, what remedies are appropriate and effective. Moreover, issues that arise in the context of health care cannot be understood or resolved by simple analogy to education, housing, or employment. Anti-discrimination law is most developed in the area of public education, where almost all action is plainly "public." Health care is characterized by public funding and private control. Public funding takes the form of publicly subsidized insurance, direct funding of specific service programs, provision of construction and education funds, and tax exemptions for capital investment in health care facilities, personal health expenditures, and not-for-profit organizations. Private decision making is influenced by technological concerns, pressures to maximize revenues, the need for financial stability, and the relative importance of personal preferences growing out of the fact that health services are, after all, intimate personal services.

BOUNDARIES OF THIS INQUIRY

This study was intended to document the extent to which race/ethnicity and handicaps are associated with disparities in people's ability to obtain care and in the amount and quality of care they receive. Disparities in the receipt of services are particularly important to question when they do not appear to reflect differences in need.[1]

The study was also to seek possible explanations for such disparities, which may result from such factors as differences in geographic proximity to services, in beliefs about health and about the value and appropriateness of medical care, or in ability to pay. Of particular concern in a civil rights context are disparities resulting from impediments to care because of racial/ethnic or handicapping factors.

The study was not intended to prove that discrimination exists or to recommend enforcement actions against it. Similarly, no attempt was made to limit the discussion to matters that clearly involve illegal discrimination or a discriminatory intent.[2] The legal definition of discrimination is not settled and will emerge only from the decisions of the courts when confronted with particular cases and sets of facts. To date, there has been very little civil rights litigation on the health care matters examined in this report.

The examination of disparities among groups may itself need explanation, since appropriate medical care must be defined by physicians and patients, in part, in terms of factors that vary from patient to patient. Each patient has unique characteristics; to see patients as individuals rather than as members of classes is an admirable ideal in medicine. Yet, experiences take on meaning from their context; data on patterns of care are essential if we are to separate random events from systematic occurrences. The examination of variations in rates and the factors associated with those variations can tell a great deal about the operation of systematic factors that may be linked with such patient characteristics as race or handicaps. It is important to know if a policy or practice that limits a person's ability to obtain needed care is focused on, for example, a particular racial group or whether it encompasses a larger grouping (for example, poor people) that contains disproportionate numbers of persons from that racial group. Only through examination of rates and sources of variation can such factors be disentangled.

It was recognized at the outset of this study that the subject matter was broad and that a variety of factors contribute to disparities in health care. This report identifies problem areas, tentatively examines hypotheses about possible causes, and recommends future data-gathering activities that would allow more definitive conclusions and policy recommendations to be reached. Selectivity was necessary because of limitations on on the availability of both evidence and the resources to review it. For example, no examination of the Indian Health Service was attempted. The problems raised by hospital closures and relocations were largely excluded from the study at the request of the OCR, which had other activities under way on that topic.[3] Only limited attention was given to issues that arise in psychiatric care.

This report is based primarily on the committee's review of the relevant research and statistical literature on health care, its attempts to identify data sources and methodological approaches of potential usefulness, and its review of the responsibilities of the OCR and past civil rights enforcement activities. In some instances the committee sought and obtained, particularly from the National Center for Health Statistics, new analyses of existing data that helped to shed light on particular questions. In addition, by means of a hearing in Washington, a series of briefings at a meeting of the committee in Los Angeles, and through correspondence with many organizations, the committee obtained the views of persons who have been actively engaged in concerns about the health care of the groups on which this study focuses.

SUMMARY

The major theme of this report is the extent to which race/ethnicity or handicaps affect whether and where people obtain medical care and the quality of that care. The committee reached the general conclusion that race is associated with differences in the use of health services and that these differences do not mirror differences in need. The causal relationships behind these associations are complex and poorly documented. However, existing data are too incomplete and contradictory to provide either a full picture of disparities or clear explanations of racial and ethnic patterns of health services use. With regard to handicapped populations, there are not only serious deficiencies in data, but criteria are lacking for judging whether unwarranted disparities exist. Available evidence fails to provide an adequate picture of services obtained by those with handicapping conditions. At the same time, the state of the law is uncertain with respect to application of civil rights laws to the health care scene. Studies and legal tests that would clarify these matters are needed. The following chapters include recommendations for data collection.

This report contains five chapters. The remainder of Chapter 1 sets forth the committee's findings and conclusions. Subsequent chapters provide the evidence on which the committee's conclusions rest. Chapter 2 summarizes available evidence regarding the health status and health care of racial and ethnic minorities. Chapter 3 presents a more detailed analysis of the possible explanations for one of the most striking racial discrepancies in health care: the use of nursing homes. Chapter 4 discusses the health care of handicapped persons, especially obstacles that bear on their ability to obtain needed care. Chapter 5 examines the legal approaches by which civil rights concerns can be addressed, including direct enforcement of civil rights laws by the OCR, the activities of health planning agencies, and the commitments made by institutions in obtaining Hill-Burton funds for facility construction.

Racial/Ethnic Patterns in Health Care

Chapter 2 describes evidence on the extent to which race and ethnicity affect people's need for medical care, the amount of care they receive, the sources from which they obtain care, and the quality of the care they receive. The evidence reviewed by the committee pertains in the main to blacks and, to a lesser extent, Hispanics.

There is considerable evidence that racial and ethnic factors are associated with disparities in patterns of health care. Although the data reviewed in Chapter 2 are not definitive, they clearly support the concern of many people that minority groups are still discriminated against in this country. The committee's findings include the following:

- Anecdotes abound of instances of minority patients who are seriously ill, badly injured, or in active labor being turned away from hospitals, transferred to other (public) hospitals, or subjected to long delays before care is provided. These problems appear to be most frequent for blacks in the south and for the Mexican American, immigrant, and American Indian populations of the Southwest and West. The cases may involve both patients' racial/ethnic status and their poverty and result from the application of such hospital policies as requiring advance payment under certain circumstances, refusing to accept Medicaid, not informing patients of the "free care" obligations that the hospital assumed in accepting Hill-Burton funds, not accepting patients who do not have a personal physician, requiring that poor patients complete applications for Medicaid (which may deter immigrant patients who are here under color of law but who are not U.S. citizens), and attempting to determine the immigration status of patients and to transfer to Mexican hospitals patients about whom some question exists. Although the effects of such policies can be identified in particular cases, little systematic data exist to enable an overall assessment of the extent to which such factors affect the health care of minority group members.
- By a variety of measures, the average need for medical care among racial/ethnic minorities exceeds that of whites. However, notwithstanding the greater needs of these groups, they do not receive more hospitalization or physician visits than whites. Evidence from the mid-1970s suggests that federal health programs have increased poor people's ability to obtain medical care and have accomplished a reduction in some disparities in health care. However, low use of dental services among blacks and Hispanics and of nursing home use among blacks is particularly striking.
- A variety of forms of racial separation or segregation exist in American health care. There are obvious racial differences in where people obtain medical care, both with regard to physician visits and hospital use. Blacks are less likely than whites to see private physicians, regardless of income level or type of insurance. Blacks are less likely than whites to see specialists rather than general practitioners. Racially identifiable hospitals continue to exist in many large cities.
- Only scattered evidence is available regarding racial/ethnic differences in quality of medical care received. There are some anecdotal suggestions of poor-quality medical care for blacks in the South. There is evidence that the care provided to some minority groups comes from health professionals that are comparatively less well qualified. There is also less satisfaction with medical care among minority group members.

• Data limitations prevent an adequate description of racial/ethnic differences in health care and an adequate analysis of possible causes. Very little quantitative information is available on the extent of segregation in health care, how this varies by region, state, and city; and how federal policy (for example, regarding Medicaid) affects it. Racial/ethnic variables have not, with a few exceptions, been examined in the literature on medical care quality.

From these findings, the committee drew several conclusions. First, racial/ethnic patterns in health care deserve much more serious and systematic attention than they have received from researchers and governmental statistical agencies. More studies are needed that empirically examine the factors that influence the medical care decisions of minority group members. In recent years, the National Center for Health Statistics and the National Center for Health Services Research have begun to show more concern for collecting statistically valid data on separate minority groups; such data are expensive to collect because of sampling problems, yet they are of great importance if equity questions in American health care are to be assessed. The present Health Care Financing Administration (HCFA) data are so inadequate that it is virtually impossible to draw meaningful conclusions about racial/ethnic equity in the Medicaid, Medicare, and Title V programs. HCFA should exert strong efforts to improve the quality of the racial/ethnic information on beneficiaries of these crucially important federal financing programs. An agreement between HCFA and OCR in 1980 may be a first step in increasing HCFA's attention to racial and ethnic issues.

Second, in light of the evidence on racial differences in the sources of medical care, the question of racial segregation in health care, and associated questions regarding quality of health care, deserve much more attention than they have received. At present, some federal policies do not encourage racial/ethnic integration in health care. For example, policies that encourage the concentration of Medicaid patients into certain facilities contribute to racial/ethnic segregation in areas where members of some minority groups are disproportionately dependent upon Medicaid.

Third, specific attention should be given to the factors that may explain the striking racial patterns regarding dental care. The data clearly show that the need for dental care (as defined by untreated disease) is much greater among blacks than among whites and the use of dental services is much greater among whites than among blacks. The data also suggest that these trends are due to more than socioeconomic differences.

Blacks and Nursing Homes

The committee gave special attention to this topic because blacks use nursing homes at markedly lower rates than do whites. The committee believed that an assessment of the evidence that might explain this would not only be useful for its own sake, but also to illustrate the general complexities underlying racial/ethnic differences in health care. Although racial discrimination has been offered as an explanation for racial differences in the use of nursing homes, various other explanations have also been suggested, including differences in family networks and values among blacks and whites, differences in geographic proximity to nursing homes, racial differences in life expectancy, and racial differences in income.

The evidence reviewed in Chapter 3--including published studies, anecdotal observations, and testimony presented to the committee--is consistent with the hypothesis that blacks are discriminated against in nursing home admissions. Nevertheless, little direct, systematic documentation of such discrimination exists. Most of the evidence that leads the committee to conclude that racial discrimination may play a role in nursing home admissions pertains to inadequacies of competing explanations for the low rates of nursing home use among blacks. The committee found that:

- Racial differences in life expectancy do not account for the lower use of nursing homes by blacks than by whites, because the differences exist in nursing home use within age categories, particularly among persons above age 75.
- The lower rates of nursing home use among blacks are not attributable to superior health status, because there is more disability among elderly blacks than among elderly whites.
- Elderly blacks are more likely than elderly whites to reside as part of an extended family, which supports the hypothesis that family factors contribute to the relative absence of blacks in nursing homes. However, it is also possible that the living arrangements of elderly blacks are the result of, rather than the reason for, their lower nursing home use.
- Racial difference in the frequency of extended family living arrangements notwithstanding, one national survey suggests that there are only minimal racial differences among partially disabled elderly persons in the availability of persons (including non-relatives) to provide needed assistance at home. Among blacks, such persons are more likely than those among whites to reside in the same household. However, the lack of assistance at home (an obvious reason for entering a nursing home) does not appear from this survey to vary between blacks and whites and thus cannot explain the racial difference in the use of nursing homes.
- The black elderly are more likely than white elderly to be institutionalized in settings other than nursing homes, such as mental and chronic disease hospitals. This too casts doubt on the hypothesis that certain values or living arrangements that are more common among blacks than among whites lead to greater black reluctance to rely on institutions to provide needed care of the elderly. (Although good data do not exist, some observers believe that blacks, more commonly than whites, reside in unlicensed boarding facilities that meet, however poorly, some of the needs that nursing homes more often meet for whites.)

- Nursing home beds tend to be in short supply in states with relatively high proportions of blacks, which may partially account for the low rates of nursing home use among blacks. No data are available to assess the possible effects of proximity to nursing homes within metropolitan areas in influencing racial patterns of nursing home use.
- The weaker economic position of blacks and their disproportionate dependence on Medicaid must influence their use of nursing homes. The demand for nursing home beds exceeds the supply in many locales, and most nursing homes maintain a waiting list. There are important disincentives for accepting Medicaid patients, both economic (private-paying patients typically are charged more than the Medicaid payment level) and administrative (paperwork and review procedures designed to prevent unnecessary utilization). Thus, there are good reasons to expect nursing homes to discriminate against Medicaid patients, whose number is disproportionately black.
- There are large variations among states in the representation of blacks among Medicaid patients in nursing homes. In many states, blacks constitute roughly the same proportion of the Medicaid population of nursing homes as their proportion in the state's elderly, poor population. However, in several states for which data are available--most notably Mississippi, Alabama, and South Carolina--white Medicaid patients are found in nursing homes in proportions far in excess of their representation among the state's elderly poor. There is also evidence of variation from city to city in the underrepresentation of blacks in nursing homes. Such state and city variations cast further doubt on the idea that familial factors and values explain the low use of nursing homes by blacks, because it seems unlikely that black values and family structures vary greatly between such cities as Baltimore and Philadelphia. Instead, these findings suggest that, in addition to whatever discrimination exists against Medicaid patients, there is also discrimination in some states and cities against blacks within the Medicaid population.
- Nursing homes tend toward racial exclusivity in some areas, making the patient population of nursing homes either virtually all white or all black. Case studies in Baltimore and Philadelphia suggest that there may be an association between the extent of segregation in nursing homes and the extent to which blacks are underrepresented. However, no conclusions can be drawn about this association because so little systematic documentation is available about the racial exclusivity of nursing homes. Economic, social, and cultural factors undoubtedly influence people's choices of nursing homes, and racial clustering in nursing homes is not conclusive evidence of discrimination.

On the basis of this evidence, the committee concluded that there is a strong likelihood that racial discrimination is an important factor in the admission of blacks into nursing homes, though how widespread a factor is not clear. The evidence reviewed in Chapter 3--particularly concerning state variations in the underrepresentation of blacks in the Medicaid population of nursing homes and concerning patterns of racial segregation in nursing homes--also suggests a basis for focusing civil rights compliance review activities.

Because data shortcomings were apparent throughout the preparation of Chapter 3, the committee also offered some suggestions about priorities and research approaches, emphasizing the need for information about coping by persons who need nursing home care and about patterns of segregation in nursing homes and the processes that contribute to such patterns. In some cases, useful information can be obtained from existing data sources, but other questions can be answered only through the collection of new data. Data from the National Nursing Home Survey do not show a black/white differential in nursing home use below age 74; such findings may be used in establishing priorities for more detailed investigation of racial patterns in the use of nursing homes.

Health Care of Handicapped Persons

Although handicapped persons are covered by laws prohibiting discrimination in federal programs, few systematic data exist on the health care of handicapped persons that would allow for an assessment of the nature and severity of discrimination problems they face. Handicapped persons constitute a large and diverse segment of the American population. They include people with various types and degrees of permanent disabilities and people with different chronic physical and mental conditions that may require long-term therapy. In part, because of this diversity, the handicapped population is not always well understood. The concerns of handicapped people about problems of discrimination was recognized in the passage of Section 504 of the Rehabilitation Act, which prohibits discrimination against the handicapped in any program receiving federal financial assistance. The handicapped population's vulnerability to discrimination can be heightened by the fact that it includes disproportionate numbers of the poor, the black, and the elderly. Many handicapped persons are to some degree dependent upon governmental programs for meeting their needs, including their needs for health care.

There is confusion and lack of consensus about such basic matters as the meaning of "handicap" and the definition of discrimination. One unfortunate source of confusion is Section 504 itself, which defines as handicapped any person who has a "physical or mental impairment that substantially limits one or more of the person's life activities." This definition, which does not differentiate disabled persons from persons with chronic diseases, includes many persons who are not customarily regarded as handicapped (for example, alcoholics or people with chronic physical illnesses). More confusion stems from the variety of governmental programs that serve persons who are handicapped or disabled. There is little definitional coherence or consistency among these programs; features that make handicapped persons eligible for certain programs may make them ineligible for others.

There appears to be little public awareness about discrimination in the health care of handicapped persons, and there may be little consensus about what should be regarded as discrimination. Discrimination is frequently thought of as treating similarly situated persons differently; however, in the context of the medical care of handicapped persons, discrimination may mean failing to treat differently situated persons differently (for example, not having an interpreter available for a deaf patient). Even among professionals, the question of what is discriminatory may prove vexing, as in the general problem of what needs should be met through mainstream care settings (that is, care in which handicapped persons are integrated with non-handicapped persons) and what needs would better be met in specialized settings. Similarly, as efforts are made to focus scarce resources where they will produce the most benefit, the physical or mental condition of patients may increasingly be suggested as criteria of eligibility for publicly supported programs. A given amount of dollars may benefit more people if it is focused on the least severely disabled people.

An assessment of the health care of any group can only be made in comparative terms--comparison across groups, comparison across time, or comparison against ideals. A difficulty in assessing the care of handicapped persons is the lack of comparison groups. The adequacy of care received by spinal-cord-injured patients cannot be assessed, for example, by comparing the amount of care received in a period of time with the amount of care received by another group of patients. The adequacy of care of persons with particular medical or psychological needs can only be assessed in comparison with an ideal or some other independent criteria.

In considering this problem in the assessment of the health care of handicapped persons, the committee tentatively agreed that the adequacy of such care might usefully be judged on two bases, both of which are empirically difficult to apply. First, is the care provided to handicapped persons equally effective, in relation to existing knowledge, as the care received by non-handicapped persons? Second, does the care of handicapped persons unnecessarily restrict their autonomy and independence?

Because of differences in needs, a simplistic goal of equality of services makes little sense in comparing the health care of handicapped persons and the rest of the population. It is more appropriate to think in terms of equal effectiveness of care, because treatment that ignores particular needs of handicapped persons can produce unsatisfactory results. In providing care for health problems that handicapped people share with non-handicapped people, the goal of equally effective care can be approached by attention to architectural barriers, communication aids, and sensitive and knowledgeable personnel. Few data are available that address the question of whether equally effective care is provided to handicapped persons when they develop the same medical conditions (exclusive of their handicaps) as non-handicapped persons.

Most attention under Section 504 has been on issues that arise at the point of delivery of medical care, but the goal of equally effective care can also be considered in a broader context. It can be questioned whether health care needs that are unique to people with particular disabling conditions are being met as effectively, within the limits of our knowledge in biomedical and behavioral sciences, as are the acute care needs of most of the American people. The answer can be sought by considering societal priorities in allocations for various types of health care facilities and for the training of various types of health professionals and specialists, as well as by examining the types of services that are encouraged by the incentives in the reimbursement system. In all of these areas, priority appears to be on the care of persons with acute diseases rather than persons with chronic illnesses or disabilities. This probably has a profound effect on the adequacy of care received by handicapped and disabled persons, but it is doubtful whether problems of societal priorities can be addressed through the Section 504 prohibition on discrimination. However, if the particular health care needs of handicapped and disabled persons are to be met adequately, established patterns of financing and availability of facilities and personnel must be questioned. Only then will the depth of the societal commitment, manifested by the passage of Section 504, be clear.

The second criterion of care for handicapped persons--whether it promotes or hampers their independence and autonomy--is important because societal responses to their plight have too often demanded the sacrifice of independence or of dependency. The committee concluded that, as with the criteria of equal effectiveness, serious problems exist today in providing care to handicapped persons in ways that make use of their knowledge and ability and, hence, that encourage their independence. Problems range from the work disincentives that are structured into federal programs on which many handicapped persons must depend for their medical care to the failure of health care personnel to recognize and use handicapped patients' own knowledge, experience, and capabilities in the management of their medical problems.

In its examination of health care of handicapped persons, the committee identified a number of deterrents to change. One obstacle is economic; there will be additional costs associated with solving many of the problems discussed in Chapter 4. Furthermore, because many handicapped and disabled people are dependent upon government programs for their care, they are vulnerable to reductions in services in the name of cost containment. Handicapped persons are also likely to continue to face other obstacles that have an economic rationale, such as problems in obtaining health insurance, the waiting period of 29 months for disability coverage under Medicare, state variations in coverage under Medicaid, refusal of many providers to accept Medicaid, use of medical screens (to exclude potentially heavy users of services) in insurance and in prepaid health care settings, and nursing homes' discrimination against "heavy-care patients" when reimbursement levels are fixed.

Various conceptual problems complicate the task of assessing empirically the adequacy of health care of handicapped persons. For example, research on equity or fairness in health care has generally rested on the premise that need, not such factors as income or race, should determine whether a person obtains health care. Although this idea is quite applicable to the health care of handicapped persons, applying it operationally in research is problematic, except, perhaps, in some small-scale studies. It would be difficult or impossible to identify handicapped and non-handicapped populations that are equivalent in need for care and that can, thus, be meaningfully compared in terms of use of services. Some handicapping or chronic conditions (such as cystic fibrosis) produce greater mortality, morbidity, and use of health services, while other disabilities may be a secondary effect of other chronic conditions associated with the use of health services, such as blindness resulting from diabetes. Thus, it is difficult to find a common basis on which to compare the health care of the handicapped with that of other persons to find whether such care is affected by factors other than need. However, even without such comparisons, it is possible to seek to identify factors that interfere with handicapped persons' ability to obtain health care in a manner that maximizes their independence and their status as an integral part of American society.

Existing data do not allow even a minimally adequate, empirical assessment of the problems experienced by handicapped persons in seeking or obtaining health care. Data problems may also impede coordination among various programs. Available information about even such basic matters as the number and characteristics of handicapped persons in the United States has serious shortcomings that will not be corrected by data from either the 1978 Social Security Survey (because of its limitation to "work disability") or from the 1980 U.S. Census (which did not collect any relevant information). The Census provides the best opportunity to collect reliable information about populations that are small and scattered and nearly impossible to survey adequately on a sample basis. The lost opportunity of the 1980 Census should be corrected in 1990, and data should be collected that would allow an adequate description of the numbers and characteristics of handicapped persons in the United States.

The committee also recommends that the present lack of information about the health care of handicapped persons be given attention by the Department of Health and Human Services. More uniformity in definitions, units of measurement, and classification procedures are needed if a more adequate response is to be given the legal requirements in Section 504 and other federal legislation. Improvements could come by developing operational definitions for use in (a) compiling information about handicapped beneficiaries of federal programs, and (b) collecting information by surveys. Such definitions should be reasonably consistent with the definition set forth under Section 504: a physical or mental impairment that significantly limits a person in a major life activity, not just in terms of work disability. The definition should make clear that temporary impairments (acute conditions) are not included.

Much may be learned by including questions about handicaps and disabilities in large surveys. Information about the health status of handicapped persons, where they obtain their health care, how they pay for it, what problems they experience in obtaining it, their satisfaction with it, and so forth can be obtained in surveys of the general population only if measures are taken to oversample handicapped persons. Consideration should be given to developing standard questions about handicaps that can be included in any general health survey of sufficient size and be used in the presentation of results.

In addition, more specific information is needed about the sources of care of handicapped persons and the problems they face in obtaining care. To be most useful, survey instruments should reflect both the types of handicap-specific problems (such as interpreters for deaf patients) that arise in the Section 504 context and problems (such as distance from specialized facilities or lack of coverage under health insurance) that do not. Information about sources of payment for care and participation in governmental programs will also increase the usefulness of such a data-collection effort. Because of sampling problems and because handicap-specific questions might have to be included to obtain useful information about handicapped persons, studies focused on particular handicapped populations may be needed to obtain good information about health care problems.

In addition to research that would seek information from handicapped persons themselves about the problems they face in obtaining health care, more information is needed about systematic factors that may influence the care they receive. These include state variations in federally funded programs on which many handicapped persons are dependent, information about planning agencies' attention to the health care problems of handicapped persons, and the involvement of such persons in health planning activities.

The potential impact of Section 504 in addressing problems in the health care of handicapped people is still difficult to assess. Enforcement activities to date have been limited. Section 504 may prove to be of help in solving certain problems faced by handicapped persons and in increasing societal awareness of those problems. Difficulties of architectural barriers and of communication with hearing-impaired patients are covered, at least at the regulatory level, under Section 504. Practices such as the use of medical screens, the use of physical or mental criteria in determining eligibility for programs such as the Crippled Children's Program, and discrimination against heavy-care patients in nursing homes may be inconsistent with Section 504, although the economic component of these practices should be given proper recognition in policy decisions intended to be remedies.

It appears, however, that some of the most important difficulties in the health care of the handicapped persons cannot be addressed readily, if at all, under Section 504. These include the scarcity of rehabilitation personnel and facilities, limitations of health care financing programs, and stereotyping and insensitivity by some health personnel.

Anti-discrimination Enforcement in Health Care

Although the equal protection clause of the Fourteenth Amendment of the U.S. Constitution generally prohibits discrimination in governmental activities, implementation through statutes, regulations, and court decisions is required to give practical meaning to the constitutional protection for civil rights. The necessary implementing structure is not as well developed in health as in areas such as education, employment, housing, and voting rights. Title VI of the Civil Rights Act of 1964 is clearly the most prominent civil rights statute of relevance to health, even though it does not specifically mention health. Title VI prohibits racial discrimination by providers who receive federal financial funds and requires agencies to terminate aid in the event of non-compliance.

Implementing regulations issued by the Department of Health, Education, and Welfare in 1965 (and amended in 1973) prohibit the denial of services or benefits on the basis of race, color, or national origin and any form of differential or segregated treatment. These regulations make no specific reference to the obligations of health care providers, although guidelines developed in 1969 interpret the duties of such organizations in some detail. Beyond these, there are few other federal directives specifying the application of Title VI to the health care context.

Enforcement of Title VI (and Section 504 of the Rehabilitation Act) in health care is the responsibility of the Office for Civil Rights (OCR) in the Department of Health and Human Services. However, only a few monitoring and compliance review activities have taken place in health care since the efforts to end policies of explicit hospital segregation in the first years after the passage of Medicare.

In recent years, however, OCR has undertaken steps that may lead to more civil rights enforcement activities in health care. In large part this has been in response to legal actions undertaken by private advocacy groups and from individual complaints alleging discrimination by health care providers. With the splitting off of education activities into the Department of Education, the OCR staff in DHHS will presumably be devoted primarily to health, and OCR has announced ambitious plans in that regard. Clearly, the notion of civil rights in health is still evolving and will be greatly influenced by recent and future legal cases in this area. Increased enforcement activity under existing laws will begin to resolve many of the legal uncertainties that now exist. The first attempts to apply these laws to health care discrimination are so recent that their meaning and effects are not yet clear.

In recent years, OCR (and some civil rights advocates) have shown growing interest in other statutory tools that may be used to advance the interests of groups protected by civil rights laws. These tools include the Hill-Burton program for facility construction and its successor program, the more broadly mandated National Health Planning and Resources Development Act of 1974.

Although the Planning Act was not developed specifically in response to issues in the health care of minority groups, it provided for the creation of local and state planning agencies that provide a forum within which certain civil rights concerns may be addressed. To date there has been only limited explicit attention to civil rights issues within the planning program for reasons that include the limited funding and authority of planning agencies and the lack of consistent federal guidance regarding the juncture of planning and civil rights. Nevertheless, the role of planning agencies has emerged as a serious issue in major civil rights cases in Wilmington, Delaware, and New Orleans, Louisiana, and regulations proposed in 1980 more explicitly linked planning and civil rights. However, without further clarification of the civil rights responsibilities of planning agencies and strengthening of their authority, their potential role in civil rights is limited.

The Hill-Burton program of federal grants for hospital construction provides another basis for addressing certain problems that disproportionately affect minority groups. The Hill-Burton legislation requires recipients of its construction funds to meet requirements that prohibit discrimination on account of race, creed, or color (often called the "community service" requirement, since it can be interpreted as requiring access to all people who need the services of the facility and, presumably, who are able to pay for it) and provision of a reasonable amount of "uncompensated services" for persons unable to pay. For many years, no program of enforcement existed for the community service requirement. But regulations published in the 1970s interpret community service to require Hill-Burton recipients to participate in Medicare and Medicaid and not to discriminate against such patients. Court challenges to these regulations are still taking place, and no active enforcement program is under way. Thus, the importance of Hill-Burton in the civil rights context remains to be seen.

From its review of the law and past enforcement efforts, the committee concluded that such activities have been quite limited and that existing regulations are vague when applied to health care. Although more than 15 years have elapsed since the passage of the Civil Rights Act, there still remains little guidance as to its application in health care. Because it is difficult to say what policies and practices violate Title VI, both enforcement and related research activities have been inhibited. Effective enforcement has also been limited by OCR's lack of direct authority and by the past emphasis on civil rights issues in other fields, most notably education.

Further clarification and specification of the requirements of Title VI and Section 504 in health care are needed. Several policy directions that have developed out of civil rights enforcement efforts in recent years should be more widely debated and, perhaps, codified in regulations or guidelines. Examples include conclusions about physical access and availability of transportation that developed from OCR's investigation of the civil rights implications of a hospital relocation in Wilmington, Delaware; remedies for vestiges of past segregation that were developed in a Title VI investigation in New Orleans; and OCR's position on whether a showing of intent to discriminate is necessary to a finding that discrimination is occurring.

In addition, clarification is needed regarding other matters such as the Title VI responsibilities of planning agencies, the responsibilities of health facilities serving substantial numbers of non-English-speaking people, the Title VI responsibilities of facilities that plan to close or convert services, and the scope and nature of responsibilities of providers and planning agencies under Section 504 of the Rehabilitation Act. Also, past policy decisions that exempted private physicians from Title VI, even if they receive Medicare or Medicaid monies, should be reconsidered if the full intent of Title VI is to be realized.

Despite the increased resources that the creation of DHHS may bring to civil rights enforcement in health, important resource allocation decisions must be made regarding (a) relative emphases of complaint investigations and compliance reviews and (b) the scope of compliance reviews.

An examination of recent enforcement efforts and testimony before the committee forcefully demonstrates that there is no consensus on a conceptual framework for evaluating "compliance" by health care providers other than the use of aggregate measures of admissions to institutional providers itemized by racial/ethnic categories. Measures of services to those with handicaps are at an even more rudimentary stage. The committee found that there are serious shortcomings in data both for assessing compliance by health care providers and for more generally assessing overall problems in the health services provided to and/or needed by minorities and the handicapped. Such data are prerequisites to enforcement activities under present legal obligations and to the continuing process of definition as to what disparities are to be regarded as unreasonable or illegitimate in terms of civil rights laws.

The committee suggests that the OCR inventory available indicators and measures of civil rights compliance, including available and potential sources of data. Much of the information contained in this report is relevant to such an inventory.

The committee also recommends that OCR work with existing data-collection agencies, such as the National Center for Health Statistics, to specify, obtain, and analyze data that are relevant to OCR's responsibilities. Even more urgent is the need for close cooperation between OCR and the Health Care Financing Administration to develop measures and indicators that will help document patterns of underutilization and segregation in federally funded health care and to focus compliance review activities.

However, data collection alone is a hollow exercise unless further specification can be made of what constitutes civil rights non-compliance by health care providers. Such specification was outside the mandate of this committee. Data collection and analysis are useless as compliance vehicles unless they are guided by informed judgments about possible explanations for disparities in the provision of services. This report is intended to provide materials from which such judgments can be made.

Existing uncertainties and confusion in defining or measuring equity in access or quality of services, and OCR's relative lack of experience with health services, make it important that the role of OCR itself be specified more clearly. The commitment of DHHS to the development and enforcement of civil rights policies in the health care context remains unclear. The statutory and regulatory framework of several health funding and planning programs includes the authorization--sometimes the mandate--for activities that pertain to civil rights, but this authorization has not effectively translated into day-to-day activities. The reforming of OCR in the new DHHS provides an opportunity to define OCR's mandate in the health arena.

OCR cannot be an effective enforcement agency without clear and strong support by the leadership of DHHS and cooperation between the OCR and other DHHS program staff. The committee urges the secretary of DHHS to resolve the present administrative ambiguities about civil rights within the agency and to make plain the commitment to enforce the law's guarantees of non-discrimination. Of most immediate practical utility, perhaps, is the potential for the coordination of OCR data-collection and monitoring efforts with the efforts of the Health Care Financing Administration (HCFA) incident to reimbursement activities.

The ambiguities in the definitions of discrimination in health cannot, however, be completely "solved" by administrative remedies. In the future, as in the past, the impact of OCR enforcement efforts under Title VI and Section 504 will rely in large part on the judicial interpretation of whether a disparate effect, without a showing of discriminatory intent, constitutes a legal violation. This question has been a subject of substantial judicial consideration in a variety of contexts, particularly employment and education. In the health context, judicial exploration of this issue is in the most formative stages.

The guidelines issued by OCR in 1969 delineate standards on which initial judgments can be made as to whether there is a cause for concern about disparate effects, and they set out the nature of the justification that may constitute acceptable explanations for these disparities. The committee recommends that the 1969 guidelines be issued as formal regulations for DHHS, either in their present form or in a revised version that retains the essential "effects" approach to defining discrimination. While the 1969 guidelines are hardly the final word on defining discrimination in the health care field, they provide a useful place to begin the process of debate, consensus, definition, and enforcement of civil rights in the health arena. Formal proposal in the _Federal Register_ would not only make an important statement about the commitment of DHHS to the enforcement of civil rights, but would also provide the occasion for public comment by all concerned parties that would itself prompt further refinement of basic principles.

Besides civil rights enforcement _per se_, the enforcement of clarified community service and equal access obligations of Hill-Burton facilities could have an important impact on alleviating some circumstances that have led to the unequal treatment of minorities by institutional health care providers. Relatively little can be said about the specific scope of that potential, since the recent interpretation of the obligation has yet to be tested and implemented. However, it seems likely that if OCR enforces the obligation, it will encounter problems similar to the overall problems of Title VI enforcement in health care--namely, problems of defining compliance, data collection and analysis, allocating resources to various kinds of enforcement activities, and, most critically, ensuring that OCR has the support of DHHS leadership and the cooperation of DHHS program staff.

CONCLUSION

Civil rights as a notion is neither simple nor static. The law and legal mechanisms are dynamic social processes that both shape and are responsive to debate and to consensus. At the same time, the various impacts of government and private health programs on different members of the population are only beginning to be appreciated. In many areas, information is not yet being sought that will help define socially acceptable or legally unacceptable disparities in health services and health status in the United States. This report is presented as a review of available information about certain disparities relating to minorities and handicapped individuals. The committee is aware of the complexities involved both in the structure and assumptions of health care in the United States and in the development of civil rights approaches, and it hopes its report will be used as a basis for the development of a clearer approach to civil rights in health and as a discussion document for improving the health of all Americans.

REFERENCES

1. The distribution of care according to need has been used as a definition of equity in the health care literature. See, for example, Lu Ann Aday, Ronald Andersen, and Gretchen V. Fleming, Health Care in the U.S.: Equitable for Whom? (Beverly Hills, CA: Sage, 1980) p. 41. Other concepts of equity that stress merit or societal contribution, rather than need, also exist. See Gene Outka, "Social Justice and Equal Access to Health Care," pp. 79-98 in Robert Veatch and Roy Branson (eds.), Ethics and Health Policy (Cambridge, MA: Ballinger, 1976).
2. Legally, the matter of intent is of continuing controversy in civil rights law. The Supreme Court in Lau v. Nichols (44 U.S. 563 (1974)) noted that practices that have the effect of discrimination by race or national origin are barred even though no purposeful design to do so has been demonstrated. Yet the importance of intent in defining discrimination is a matter of continuing legal relevance and importance, arising in a variety of contexts, including controversies about hospital closures and relocations.
3. However, the hospital closure/relocation issue is of growing importance to the health care of minority groups, as was stressed

in testimony presented to the IOM committee by Dr. John L. S. Holloman, Jr., M.D. Alan Sager, Ph.D., in 1980 testimony before the Subcommittee on Health of the House Committee on Ways and Means, presented data showing that it is a widespread phenomenon that disproportionately affects racial minorities. This element is clear in the Wilmington hospital relocation case that is summarized in Chapter 4 of this report.

2

HEALTH CARE OF MEMBERS OF RACIAL AND ETHNIC MINORITY GROUPS

This chapter examines the extent to which people's membership in certain racial and ethnic minority groups influences whether and from whom they obtain health care. The committee found that health problems are more common among some racial/ethnic minorities than among the rest of the population, and that this fact is not fully reflected in their use of health services. This is particularly true of dental services and nursing home care. There is also considerable evidence that race and ethnicity have a strong influence on where people obtain medical care, which hospitals they use, whether they obtain care from clinics or private physicians, and the credentials of the physicians from whom they obtain care. The social processes that produce these patterns are complex, involving residential patterns, differences in socio-economic status, ethnic differences in concepts and values associated with disease and treatment, constraints and incentives that are built into federal health programs, and, possibly, discrimination. The factor of discrimination, which is particularly important in a civil rights context, is poorly understood because it has not been examined much in research or in legal actions in health care. However, the disparities reviewed in this chapter, in the committee's view, suggest that the question of discrimination in health care deserves more attention than it has received.

The focus of this review stems from questions regarding civil rights and health care. In sharp contrast to such areas as employment, housing, and education, there is little to suggest that discrimination and integration in health care have been important public policy concerns in recent years. Yet some very serious problems of possible significance under civil rights laws have been described in testimony before the committee as well as before various congressional and investigative bodies and the courts. Legal services attorneys and journalists have described incidents in which minority group patients who are seriously ill, badly injured, or in active labor have been turned away from hospitals, transferred to other (public) hospitals, or subjected to long delays before care is provided.[1] In addition, accounts of segregated health facilities occasionally still come to public attention.

Most of the incidents that have been described have occurred in private, non-profit hospitals that have a substantial federal involvement through Medicare, Medicaid, or the Hill-Burton program. (See Chapter 5 for a discussion of relevant legal issues.) Problems appear to be most serious for blacks in the South and for the Mexican-American and Indian populations of the Southwest and West. The cases generally appear to involve both patients' racial/ethnic status and their poverty or inability to pay for care. (The combination of minority status and poverty appears to be much more potent than either factor taken separately, as can be seen in the statistical evidence presented later in this chapter.) The grounds for refusing to provide care vary in these cases, but involve such hospital policies as requirements for advance payment under certain circumstances, non-acceptance of Medicaid or certain other sources of third-party payment, not informing patients of the "free care" obligations that the hospital assumed in accepting Hill-Burton funds, non-admission of patients who do not have a personal physician, requirements that poor patients complete applications for Medicaid (which may effectively deter immigrant patients who are here under color of law but who are not U.S. citizens), and attempting to determine the immigration status of patients and to transfer to Mexican hospitals patients about whom some question exists.*

The following descriptions, several of which come from a recent hearing of the U.S. Civil Rights Commission, are typical of these incidents, the outcomes of which have included babies being born in hospital parking lots, serious medical complications, and the death of patients. All of the facts in such anecdotes cannot be known with certainty. Nor is it known how common such occurrences are or how often non-minority patients have similar experiences. There is, unfortunately, little way of linking anecdotes with the more systematic data on patterns of use of health services that are reviewed later in this chapter. However, the anecdotes suggest possible explanations for some of the disparities that are reviewed in this chapter, and they are a source of serious concern to persons working actively on behalf of the rights and welfare of minority groups. The committee, therefore, decided that the more systematic presentation of data should be preceded by some of the anecdotes that prompted the concerns that led to this study.

---

*Because of the complexity of immigration laws, uneducated immigrants, even if they are in the country legally, may be intimidated and deterred from seeking care by hospitals' posting signs stating that they cooperate with the Immigration and Naturalization Service, by requirements that the patient complete forms (such as Medicaid applications) that are to be sent to the government, and by hospital efforts to determine their legal status. The latter practice may be questionnable, both from a legal standpoint[2] and from the standpoint of the proper purpose and mission of a hospital.

A young black woman in Memphis, Tennessee, suffering from a ruptured ectopic pregnancy, was refused admission at one private hospital that did not take Medicaid patients and was refused by a second private facility on grounds that the hospital did not take Medicaid patients for "female problems." At a public hospital facility she was informed that she would be seen, but only after the staff had treated a number of cases they considered to be more serious in nature than hers. . . . In March 1979, a 29-year-old Mexican-American woman and her baby died of a ruptured uterus in a rural part of Texas. Two hospitals had turned away this acutely ill eight-month pregnant woman for inability to pay. Similarly, Ysidro Aguinagas, an 11-month-old Hispanic baby, died in December 1978 after being denied admission to a public hospital in Dimmitt, Texas, despite the fact that the hospital was a Hill-Burton facility and publicly financed. The baby would not be admitted without a $450 deposit. Since the parents were without a $450, deposit they left the facility to seek other sources of care, but the baby died en route.[3]

On August 1, 1976, Mrs. Carolyn Payne, a 21-year-old black resident of Holly Springs, Mississippi, delivered her own baby in the front seat of a truck after the emergency room of the Marshall County Hospital had refused admission. The Marshall County Hospital is a 60-bed county facility in Holly Springs, built with federal Hill-Burton funds, and supported by state and county health funds.[4]

Spanish-speaking citizens of Mexican descent are often presumed to be illegal or undocumented persons when they arrive for services in hospitals in southern California. A November 1979 newsletter reports an incident wherein an Hispanic man, conscious and speaking Spanish, arrived at an emergency room at 7 p.m. for treatment of stab wounds suffered in an attack. No doctor arrived until 8:30. Upon arrival, the doctor inquired about insurance for the patient and whether the patient was in the country legally. The wife, also Spanish speaking and monolingual, could not satisfactorily answer these questions. By 10 p.m. that evening, three hours after his arrival, the patient died. He had been inadequately treated. He was a U.S. citizen.[5]

In some of the cases, questions exist both about the facts and the state of the law that can only be resolved in the appropriate legal or administrative settings. The purpose of this chapter is neither to validate specific complaints nor to recommend how the legal and financial questions that arise in these situations should be resolved, but to provide a larger context within which certain social policy questions regarding equity or fairness in health care can be considered and to suggest some means by which disparities can better be understood.

The primary approach used in this chapter is the review of the research and statistical literature on the health care of racial and ethnic minority groups. However, the statistical information reviewed in this chapter does not permit a direct assessment of how common unfortunate incidents like those described above are. The examples that have come to light generally have not been through the organized data-collection activities of researchers or governmental statistical agencies. It is most difficult to link individual stories with aggregate statistics. Yet, to understand the meaning of any particular incident, such as might occur between a patient and a hospital admitting office, it is essential to understand into what pattern the incident might fit.

While much of this chapter is concerned with racial/ethnic patterns in health care, it should be recognized that such patterns may have a variety of causes. However, the absence of racial differences in health care, except where there are differences in need for care, would be strong evidence that no widespread patterns of discrimination exist. It is significant, therefore, that the committee found that racial and ethnic factors continue to be important in health care. This and the following chapter examine racial/ethnic aspects of several segments of the health care system, such as physician visits, hospitalization, nursing homes, and dental care. The analysis is concerned with questions regarding (1) whether racial and ethnic factors affect people's ability to obtain needed care, (2) the extent of racial separation in health care, and (3) whether race and ethnicity affect the quality of medical care received.

With regard to the first of these questions, there are indications that racial/ethnic differences in the use of services have been greatly reduced since the mid-1960s, although dental and nursing home care continue to be strongly related to race. To date, most governmental concern with racial/ethnic aspects of obtaining health care has been with trying to assure the availability of medical care to people who, because of poverty or place of residence, have not found care available. As noted in this chapter, some successes have been achieved, although questions of equity continue to arise.

The second set of concerns pertains to patterns of racial/ethnic separation or segregation in the health care system and the processes and factors that contribute to such patterns. Integration has not been an important consideration underlying governmental health policy. Indeed, governmental policies, such as the initial use of Hill-Burton money to construct segregated facilities or, more recently, reimbursement policies that lead to the concentration of Medicaid patients in certain institutions, may be an important cause for a tendency toward segregation in health care.

In the view of the committee, any examination of racial/ethnic differences in medical care must consider differences not only in the use of medical services but also in the source of medical care. Few carefully documented historical studies exist of racial patterns in health care, and most historical accounts of the medical care of blacks in the United States focus on issues that pertain to medical manpower rather than the behavior of patients. Thus, most accounts have emphasized the black physician's role, barriers faced in their obtaining hospital admitting privileges, and the development of racially segregated health care facilities by law and custom. In some locales, hospitals either refused to treat black patients or withheld admitting privileges from black physicians, which led to the establishment of black hospitals.[6]

Only with the landmark Simkins v. Moses H. Cone Memorial Hospital decision regarding a segregated Hill-Burton hospital in Greensboro, North Carolina, was an explicit policy of promoting segregation abandoned within the U.S. Public Health Service.[7] That was in 1963, the year before the Civil Rights Act was passed with its Title VI prohibition on racial discrimination in any program receiving federal financial assistance. Even one year after the passage of the Act, a U.S. Civil Rights Commission study found no discernable pattern of compliance in two-thirds of the hospitals surveyed. The subsequent enactment of the Medicare program made most hospitals and nursing homes potential recipients of federal funds. The Department of Health, Education, and Welfare then established an office to screen hospital applicants to see that policies of discrimination were not in effect and, after a four-month review process, reported that 3,000 hospitals that had previously practiced discrimination or segregation had come into compliance with Title VI.[8] Although the effectiveness of the screening procedure came under subsequent criticism by the U.S. Civil Rights Commission and others,[9] it was clear that an era was at an end, at least with regard to medical institutions in the United States, most of which received federal funds and were covered by the Civil Rights Act. (The practice of medicine in the offices of physicians was not directly affected by Title VI because of a DHEW determination that the indirect method through which they received federal dollars from Part B of Medicare did not constitute federal involvement sufficient to bring them under the authority of the Civil Rights Act.)

The third set of concerns addressed in this chapter pertains to whether there are racial/ethnic differences in quality of medical care. The research literature on quality of medical care has devoted only limited attention to the race/ethnicity of patients as a factor that might influence quality of care, although the committee identified some approaches that are potentially useful in this regard.

A recurrent problem encountered in this review concerns the availability of data. In many studies, minority groups are not represented in sufficient numbers to allow separate conclusions to be drawn about them.* The smaller and more dispersed the minority, the less adequate are the data. Frequently, the problem of small numbers leads to the grouping of diverse populations. Hayes-Bautista's

---

*It should be noted, however, that this chapter, which emphasizes racial rather than ethnic patterns, does not fully reflect the availability of information about other ethnic groups because of limitations in time and resources.

discussion of the diverse groups that are sometimes labeled "Hispanics" and of the confusion that is thus injected into public policy provides one example.[10] However, in many studies and sources of data, the lumping together of minority groups poses greater problems than considering as one population ("Hispanics") the Raza of the Southwest, Haitians and Cubans in Miami, and Puerto Ricans in New York. In many studies data are presented only for "whites" and "others" or "non-whites." Important differences can be obscured by combining non-white groups in which poor health is relatively common with groups (e.g., Chinese or Japanese Americans) whose health status may be better than that of other "white" Americans.

Sensitivity to all of these problems is reflected in recent reforms in governmental statistical policy and an effort to standardize a feasible set of racial and ethnic categories in all federal data-collection efforts. In recent years the virtual absence of health care data about many ethnic groups has begun to be addressed through procedures designed to provide representative samples of sufficient size of ethnic minorities. Such data are valuable in two senses: they are costly to obtain and there is no substitute for them. At present, however, the data needed to adequately assess many racial/ethnic differences in health status and use of medical services simply do not exist.

Another problem with the available information is the difficulty of disentangling causal processes underlying patterns of use of health services. Ethnicity is always characterized by particular values, beliefs, and patterns of behavior. Behavior in matters pertaining to health is a frequently cited example. Assessing the impact of ethnically linked beliefs and values is beyond the scope of this report, although some attention is given to this matter in the next chapter. Clearly, an important challenge in health care is providing care in ways that are compatible with the needs of ethnic groups. Communication problems represent the most obvious manifestation of this problem. However, the impact of ethnic cultures on health behavior and the associated responses of health providers have not been examined in this report.

HEALTH STATUS AND HEALTH CARE

Racial and ethnic differences in health status have long been recognized in the United States. Apparent inadequacies in medical care have been the object of attention in governmental programs directed at poor people and residents of areas where medical resources are scanty. The Department of Health, Education, and Welfare's (DHEW) annual compendium of information, Health United States: 1979, notes that "in general, the health status of minorities has improved during recent years, and their use of health services has increased."[11] In Health and the War on Poverty, Davis and Schoen observed that "poor people's access to medical care has increased remarkably [in the decade 1965-75] . . . steady progress has been made--particularly in those kinds of poor health that are the most prevalent among poor people and those that are most sensitive to improved medical care."[12] Finally, in their introduction to Aday, Andersen, and Fleming's massive empirical study, Health Care in the U.S., Rogers and Aiken observe that:

> The findings are encouraging, and the country has made progress since the 1960s. . . . They show that we have found ways of getting more people into the health system at levels of use that seem more commensurate with their needs than heretofore. Every subpopulation group studied has better access to medical services today [1976] than in 1963 or 1970, and in some instances the improvements have been dramatic. . . . Significant improvement for blacks is evident. The study also shows that contrary to popular opinion, most Americans (88%) seem generally satisfied with their medical care.[13]

Important qualifications, however, were attached to all of these statements. The Health United States: 1979 statement about progress is followed by the observation that "many measures indicate that the health status of minorities is not as good as that of the white majority."[14] Davis and Schoen warn that "much remains to be done. The gap [between the poor and others] has been narrowed, but not eliminated."[15] Rogers and Aiken qualify their summary of progress with the observation that 26 million people still have difficulty obtaining appropriate medical care.[16] In addition, the medical care situation of many poor people may have begun to worsen under the economic conditions of the late 1970s in ways that statistics are just beginning to show. Data from the Medicaid program, for example, show that the number of Medicaid recipients declined from 24,600,000 in 1976 to 21,600,000 in 1980.[17] Without financial access to health care, it may be anticipated that the health status of people who were formerly eligible for Medicaid will decline.

INDICATORS OF HEALTH STATUS

The medical care system cannot be held entirely responsible for the many differences in health status within a society. The causes of poor health are complex and cannot be explained by statistics alone. However, measures of health status can provide an indicator of progress that remains to be achieved and are also an essential prerequisite to intelligent interpretation of differences in the use of services.

Measures of Mortality

The most recent figures from the National Center for Health Statistics continue to show the existence of substantial racial/ethnic variations in mortality. The 1970 age-adjusted death rates show whites (6.8

deaths per year per 1,000 population) in an intermediate position between the high rates for blacks (10.4) and "American Indians and Alaska Natives" (8.2), and the low rates for Chinese Americans (4.9) and Japanese Americans (3.3).[18] There has been little change in either black or white rates since 1950, whereas the other three groups have all shown significant declines in mortality.[19] Similar racial/ethnic differences are seen in life expectancy figures, which show white life expectancy to exceed black life expectancy by four to five years,[20] whereas the life expectancy for Japanese and Chinese Americans appears to exceed white life expectancy.[21] Available data for Hispanic populations, though somewhat dated and incomplete, suggests a mortality level that falls between rates for blacks and whites.[22]

Racial differences in infant mortality rates remain pronounced. Substantial declines occurred for all racial/ethnic groups between 1950 and 1977 in infant mortality, neonatal mortality, and post-natal mortality rates.[23] Rates for Chinese Americans and Japanese Americans began and remained lower than rates for whites. The infant mortality rate for American Indians showed a dramatic reduction over this period, beginning at three times the white rate (82 per thousand live births versus 27 for whites in 1950) and moving to only slightly higher (15.6) than the white rate (12.3) in 1977. (By contrast, the post-natal mortality rate for American Indians remained at twice the white rate in 1977.) For blacks, even though substantial improvements in these mortality rates occurred in this period, rates in 1977 remained approximately twice the white rate for infant mortality (23.6 vs. 12.3), neonatal mortality (16.1 vs. 8.7), and post-natal mortality (7.6 vs. 3.6).[24] Among Hispanics, there is some evidence of infant mortality rates that are elevated above rates for whites, but the data are for very limited geographic areas, and some are dated.[25]

A difficulty in using such gross measures of health status is that they reflect many social, economic, and cultural factors, and, thus, they cannot be interpreted as unambiguous indicators of differences in the adequacy of health care of different racial/ethnic groups. Yet the rapid changes in the infant mortality rates (particularly for American Indians) demonstrate that infant mortality is subject to dramatic improvements. Furthermore, black infant mortality rates do not stand at a uniformly high level, but show considerable variation from place to place. Figures for 1973-74 showed a range of from 17.2 in the fringe areas of large cities in the western United States to a rate of 32.7 in the non-urbanized South.[26] By states, the most recent data show black infant mortality rates to vary from under 20 per 1,000 live births in Massachusetts and Washington to almost 30 per 1,000 in Illinois (and the District of Columbia).[27] Thus, it is clear that the high rate of black infant mortality is not immutable.

More generally, black mortality exceeds white mortality for most important causes of death in the United States--for major cardiovascular diseases, for cancer, for diabetes mellitus, and for accidents and homicide,[28] as well as for diseases such as influenza, pneumonia, and cirrhosis of the liver.[29] Yet mortality data seldom, if ever, mirror incidence data on how many people fall sick each year. Thus, such data cannot be interpreted as a sound measure of racial differences in the incidence of these diseases. Nor can such mortality data be used uncritically as an indicator of racial differences in medical care because mortality rates are affected by many other factors.

However, some indications of possible differences in medical care for different populations may come from data on variations in both incidence and mortality rates for a disease. For instance, the National Cancer Institute (NCI) collects data on the incidence of diagnosed cancer, the stage of disease at diagnosis, modes of treatment used, and 5- and 10-year survival rates. The overall incidence of cancer (total of all sites) is higher for blacks (318.8 per 100,000 population) than for whites (297.7), although the relative rates of incidence vary markedly from site to site.[30] (Thus, for example, breast cancer is more common in whites, while prostate cancer is more common in blacks.) The NCI data also show that for most sites cancer in whites is more likely to be localized at diagnosis than is cancer in blacks.[31] This suggests either that blacks do not obtain medical attention as early in the course of the disease as do whites or that the diagnosis of cancer is not made as early in medical evaluation of blacks as of whites. Data are not available to enable a choice between these explanations or to explain why either type of delay occurs.

The NCI data contain other information that may show the effects of racial differences in health care. Five-year survival rates for most cancer sites are lower for blacks than for whites.[32] This appears to reflect more than early diagnosis among whites because the racial difference in survival persists even when the survival rates under comparison are hospitalized patients whose cancer was localized at diagnosis.[33] The rate at which blacks develop cancer is 9 percent higher than that for whites, but the mortality rate for blacks is 30 percent higher than that for whites.[34] Although differences in medical care are not the only possible explanation for racial differences in cancer survival, and serious questions can be raised about the representativeness of the NCI data, particularly with regard to blacks,[35] the possibility that cancer survival data reflect racial differences in adequacy of medical care cannot be ignored.[36]

Similarly, racial differences in mortality from diabetes mellitus are much larger than racial differences in the incidence of the disease.[37] Again, the extent to which differences in medical care play a role cannot be assessed with existing evidence.

Measures of Morbidity

Some indication of racial/ethnic differences in the need for medical care can be gained through an examination of differences in health status, both as these are reflected in data about the incidence or prevalence of various diseases and in people's self-evaluations of their own health status. Information about the incidence or prevalence of different diseases is available from several sources--from national studies conducted by the National Center for Health Statistics, from data on reportable diseases collected by the Center for Disease Control, and through epidemiological studies conducted within particular geographic areas.

The prevalence of a large number of serious diseases is higher among blacks than among whites. Data from the U.S. National Health Survey show that, on average, blacks are much more likely than whites to report that they have diabetes, hypertension, and cerebrovascular disease, while the Center for Disease Control's data on syphilis, gonorrhea, and tuberculosis show rates much higher for blacks than whites.[38] NCI data show that cancer is more prevalent among blacks than among whites.[39] For some other diseases, such as heart disease, asthma, and some skin diseases, there is no great variation by race.[40] For some conditions, such as bronchitis, arthritis and synovitis, eczema and dermatitis, and some digestive diseases, available statistics show that rates for whites are higher than for blacks.[41]

Also relevant to the need for medical care is fertility; the birthrate is substantially higher among blacks (22 live births per 1,000 population) than among whites (14 per 1,000).[42]

The piecemeal morbidity data that exist on Hispanics suggest that a variety of diseases may be more prevalent for them than for the majority of the white population. This was true for a variety of reportable diseases (e.g., amoebic dysentery, hepatitis, measles, mumps, syphilis, tuberculosis) in Los Angeles during the early 1970s.[43] There is also some evidence of elevated morbidity and mortality associated with drug and alcohol abuse in the Puerto Rican population of New York.[44] On the other hand, studies using carefully drawn samples in Alameda County, California, show the Chicano population there to have lower rates of chronic conditions, disability, and symptoms than either whites or blacks.[45]

Measures of Health Status

Existing epidemiological evidence about the incidence or prevalence of specific diseases, though useful for many purposes, provides only a limited overall picture of racial/ethnic differences in health status. Such data are usually based either on very limited geographic areas or on reported cases that, for a variety of reasons, may not give a wholly accurate picture. (For example, people who do not seek medical care will not be counted, a factor of considerable importance if the data are to be used as indicators of whether needs for medical care are being met.)

A different approach, commonly used in household surveys, is to inquire about people's own assessments of their health status. Although such data provide a useful health indicator, they also have obvious weaknesses. Considerable evidence exists that people's perceptions about their present health status are affected by many factors (including cultural factors and their own previous health status).[46] Furthermore, people who have obtained inadequate health care in the past may have different perceptions of when discomfort signals illness, and they may also be unaware of (and, hence, unable to report) some conditions.[47] Nevertheless, self-reports of health status provide an important basis of comparison of the general health of large segments of the population.

In general, self-reports of health status show that black and Hispanic populations are more likely than whites to think they have health problems. Table 1, from the National Health Interview Survey conducted by the National Center for Health Statistics, presents data on racial, ethnic, and income differences in self-reported health status, limitation of activity, restricted-activity days, and bed days.[48] The relationship between health status and income is apparent in Table 1. In addition, within the two income categories, most of these measures show the health status of whites to be better than the other two groups, although the differences are neither large nor internally consistent.

The differences in health status are particularly pronounced in some categories of persons who are most likely to be eligible for governmental health care programs (a category of special interest in a study prompted by civil rights concerns). Health Interview Survey data show that among elderly, low-income people, the health status of blacks is markedly worse than that of whites; the national picture for Hispanics is more mixed, with rates on some measures similar to whites.[49] However, studies in cities such as New York, San Antonio, and Los Angeles suggest that the health status of such categories as "Spanish origin" or "Mexican-American" may be markedly worse than whites.[50] The poor health status of elderly black persons as compared to elderly white persons has been confirmed in other national studies as well as in local studies in Los Angeles and New York.[51]

For children, there are some major racial/ethnic differences. Large racial differences in mortality characterize the youngest age categories. These decrease with age, and among teenagers, black mortality rates are only slightly higher than rates for whites.[52] This is partially explained, however, by the greater frequency of accidental death among white teenagers; black teenagers are one-and-a-half times more likely as whites to die from disease. Parental* assessments of the health status of their children are consistent with these data. White parents are more likely than black or "Spanish" parents to assess the health of their children as "excellent," and they are less likely to assess their children's health as "fair or poor."[53] These differences are true in both families with incomes less than $10,000 and in higher-income families. Paradoxically, fewer disability days and bed days are reported for black children than for whites.[54] The National Center for Health

---

*In some instances, assessments in this household survey may have been by adults other than parents of children whose health status was being described.

Table 1. SELECTED HEALTH STATUS MEASURES, BY RACE/ETHNICITY AND INCOME, 1976-77

Income, Age, and Race or Ethnicity	Population in Thousands	Persons With Self-assessed Health Status As Fair or Poor	Persons With Limitation of Activity	Restricted-Activity Days[1]	Bed Days[2]
All Incomes[3]		Percent of Population		Number per Person per Year	
Black	23,066	19.1	14.6	20.7	8.9
Hispanic	11,913	12.8	9.1	16.7	7.8
White	160,129	11.0	14.0	17.6	6.6
Less Than $10,000					
Black	11,961	23.5	19.2	25.1	10.5
Hispanic	5,681	17.2	12.0	21.3	9.9
White	44,555	19.5	23.8	26.2	9.8
$10,000 or More					
Black	8,363	11.9	8.1	14.7	6.6
Hispanic	5,122	8.0	5.8	11.9	5.5
White	102,809	6.9	9.6	13.7	5.1

NOTE: The categories white, black, and Hispanic are mutually exclusive.

[1]Includes bed days, work-loss days, school-loss days, and other restricted-activity days.
[2]Bed days are a subgroup of restricted-activity days.
[3]Includes those for whom income was unknown.

SOURCE: Division of Health Interview Statistics, National Center for Health Statistics. Data from the Health Interview Survey.

Statistics, the source of these data, speculates that the apparent discrepancy between the parental assessments of children's health status, and the reported disability days and bed days, may be due to white children's greater access to medical attention (perhaps by telephone), which results in their being told more frequently than blacks to reduce or limit their activities.[55] This interpretation is consistent with data on physician visits by children (reviewed later in this chapter) and on available information about the health status of children.

An earlier national survey showed the reported incidence of acute conditions for persons under 17 years of age to be considerably higher for whites (270 conditions per 100 persons in 1973) than for others (169 conditions per 100 persons).[56] Still, the overall picture regarding racial/ethnic differences in the health of children is not completely clear. (Much more information about child health is summarized in the report of the Select Panel on Child Health Promotion.[57])

USE OF MEDICAL SERVICES

Although the following sections examine statistics on the use of medical services, the limitations of such data should be acknowledged at the outset. Although some promising attempts have been made, it is difficult to link such statistics with measures of need for care. Thus, there is a tendency for all physician visits, for example, to be treated as equivalent, although there may be very little need for some visits, and other visits may be generated by improper patient care at the first visit. How aggregate utilization statistics are affected by such complexities is largely unknown.

A different kind of problem arises because of the inevitable lags in data systems, a factor that is particularly important in times of rapid change. Racial and ethnic minorities that contain disproportionate numbers of poor people are differentially dependent upon compensatory institutions and programs that have been established to take care of the poor. The existence of compensatory institutions in times of growing budgets in public and municipal services is quite a different matter than in times of economic stress. Some governmental services affect most of the population--road repairs, police and fire services, and so forth--and cuts are felt across a wide segment of the population. By contrast, most governmental health programs affect relatively narrow segments of the population, making it possible to target the groups that will be affected by cuts in services. Thus, the groups that are dependent upon these programs are peculiarly vulnerable to cuts in governmental support. Since most available data on the use of health services are three to five years old, they probably do not fully reflect the current status of the health care of minority groups and, more generally, poor people.

Ambulatory Care

Visits to physicians provide a basic measure of the receipt of health care services and have been examined in national surveys conducted by the National Center for Health Statistics (NCHS) and the Center for Health Administration Studies (CHAS) at the University of Chicago. Data from both sources in the mid-1970s show a narrowing or elimination of earlier racial/ethnic differences in such matters as the interval since the last physician visit, having seen a physician in the previous year, and the number of physician visits in the previous year.[58] NCHS and CHAS data on racial/ethnic differences regarding the latter two of these measures are shown on Table 2. At the most aggregate levels, racial/ethnic differences are relatively small. However, data from the more narrowly defined ethnic samples examined in the CHAS

Table 2. PHYSICIAN VISITS, BY RACE/ETHNICITY AND INCOME

	NCHS 1976-77[1]			CHAS 1976[2]		
Number of Physician Visits Per Year	All	$10,000 & Above	Below $10,000	All	Above Poverty Level	Below Poverty Level
White[3]	5.0	4.8	5.6	4.1	4.1	4.1
Black	4.6	4.3	5.0	3.1[5] 4.4[6]	2.9[5] 4.5[6]	3.2[5] 4.3[6]
Hispanic[4]	4.2	4.0	4.5	3.5	4.3	2.9
Percent of Persons with One or More Physician Visits in Past Year						
White[3]	76	77	76	77	77	73
Black	74	77	74	65[5] 77[6]	67[5] 78[6]	64[5] 75[6]
Hispanic[4]	69	71	69	65	74	56

[1]Data from National Center for Health Statistics (NCHS). DHEW, Health United States, 1979 (Washington, D.C.: Goverment Printing Office, 1980) pp. 40-42.

[2]Data from Center for Health Administration Studies (CHAS), University of Chicago. Lu Ann Aday, Ronald Andersen, and Gretchen V. Fleming, Health Care in the U.S.: Equitable for Whom? (Beverly Hills, CA: Sage, 1980) pp. 102-106.

[3]"White" in the CHAS data does not include the "Spanish-heritage, Southwest" sample.

[4]CHAS data are from a sample of persons defined as "Spanish-heritage, Southwest."

[5]Data from sample of southern blacks not residing in Standard Metropolitan Statistical Areas (SMSAs).

[6]Data on "non-whites" other than those included in the sample of southern blacks not in SMSAs.

study show more substantial racial/ethnic variations. Lower rates of physician visits among rural southern blacks also have been reported in community studies.[59]

There are some substantial racial/ethnic differences in the number of physician visits per patient in the previous year. Fewer physician visits are reported by persons from minority groups. These differences largely reflect differences in the proportion of people who had not seen a physician at all. That is, among persons who had seen a physician the previous year, racial/ethnic differences in the average number of physician visits were smaller in magnitude; in all groups compared, the average number of physician visits for persons who had seen a physician at all was between 4.4 and 5.8.[60] Thus, it appears that, on average, those racial/ethnic barriers that are seen most clearly to exist operate in a way that affects initial physician visits (that is, whether people see a doctor at all) more than follow-up visits.

Among children, although differences in use of physician services have narrowed considerably as a result of a variety of federal programs, small racial differences still exist, as Dutton's review of the most recent information available through the Health Interview Survey conducted by the National Health Statistics shows.[61] White children had more visits to physicians (4.3 per year) than did non-white children (2.9) in 1977, and 3 to 6 percent more non-white children than white children did not see a physician at all during that year.[62] In an attempt to determine whether such figures mean white physician use is too high or non-white use is too low, Kovar reanalyzed data from the Health Interview Survey to determine the extent to which children fell below a medically defined standard of adequate numbers of physician visits.* Based on 1975-76

---

*The same unpublished data from the 1978 Health Interview Survey also show the racial difference in source of care (within different income categories) to be more pronounced in metropolitan areas (where more than two-thirds of the white population and three-fourths of the black population reside) than in non-metropolitan areas. Among metropolitan blacks below 150 percent of the poverty level, only 44 percent (compared with 63 percent of whites in the same category) report their usual source of care to be an office-based physician, and more than 26 percent (compared with 10 percent of whites) report an outpatient department or emergency room as the usual source of care.[66] Similar findings have been reported among the black and Puerto Rican populations of New York, and Weaver reports a 1969 study in Orange County, California, which found that, although English-speaking whites and Mexican Americans expressed similar preferences for receiving care from private physicians or hospitals, Mexican Americans received care at a public health facility four times more often.[67] Weaver attributes this tendency to Mexican Americans' previous negative experiences with English-speaking medical personnel, the presence of Spanish-speaking personnel in the public health facility, and the perception by English-speaking patients that the facility was a "Mexican" hospital.

data, 13 percent of white children had inadequate numbers of physician visits, compared with 19 percent of black children and 16 percent of others.[63] Thus, by a variety of measures, small but consistent differences exist in the amount of physician care received by white and non-white children.

Large-scale studies that examine racial/ethnic differences in the medical care of people with equivalent levels of medical need are scarce. One approach is to examine the medical care of persons whose needs can be considered roughly equivalent because they have similar medical conditions. Data from the National Ambulatory Medical Care Survey show that, although the prevalence of diabetes mellitus among "black and all other" women is 39 percent higher than for white women, the rate of visits to physicians' offices (per 1,000 population) for this condition is 27 percent higher for the former group than for white women.[64] The prevalence of hypertension is more than 82 percent higher among "black and all other" women than among white women, whereas the rate of visits to physicians' offices for the condition is virtually identical in the two groups.[65] These comparisons, however, are based only on visits to physicians' offices, not on all physician-patient encounters for these conditions and, thus, probably do not provide an accurate picture of overall racial differences in medical care for these conditions.

Prenatal care is a topic for comparison of racial differences in care for groups (in this case, pregnant women) that are to some degree comparable in terms of need. There is a more than 100 percent difference between whites and blacks in infant mortality. Although the causal factors underlying low birth weight are not well understood,[68] prenatal care in pregnancy has played a major role in the overall downward trend in infant mortality in the United States in recent decades. By all measures, blacks on average receive less-adequate prenatal care than whites. For example, in 1975, among blacks more than 10 percent of the live births were to women who received either late (initiated in third trimester) care or none at all, compared with 5 percent of whites.[69] Racial differences are present in all educational categories and are evident as well when illigitimate births are excluded.[70] (However, illegitimate births among both black and white women are preceeded by similarly low levels of prenatal care.[71] The low level of care for this category may be partially due to the fact that in 19 states poor women who will become eligible for Medicaid--by means of Aid to Dependent Children--after their first baby is born cannot receive services through Medicaid before the baby is born.) Whites averaged more than two more prenatal visits than blacks.[72]

Regionally, racial differences in prenatal care are most pronounced in the urban Northeast and least pronounced in the West.[73] However, it appears that the "Spanish heritage" population of the Southwest is a group that is relatively unlikely to see a physician during the first three months of pregnancy,[74] findings that have been confirmed by data from California.[75]

Another approach to examining whether there are racial differences in the relationship between medical care and medical need has been developed in the studies conducted through the Center for Health Administration Studies (CHAS) at the University of Chicago. Persons surveyed were asked about their medical care and about symptoms and days of disability. From this information, two indices (known as the use-disability ratio and the symptoms-response ratio) were constructed that incorporate measures of both medical care and need for medical care.[76] While both of these measures have limitations,[77] they are amenable to use in population-based surveys, and since 1963 these measures have shown that wide income and racial differences exist in medical care.[78] By contrast, the 1976 CHAS survey showed that earlier racial/ethnic differences had either disappeared or that, in terms of their self-reports of disability and symptoms, blacks were receiving more medical care than whites.[79] At the same time, the credence given to these measures must be tempered both by the methodological problems mentioned earlier and by other uncertainties in their use and interpretation. (One such uncertainty, as Dutton notes, is seen in the fact that different analyses of the same data from the 1976 survey have shown that large income differences exist in the use-disability ratio (number of physician visits per 100 disability days) and that no differences exist, apparently depending on what method is used to standardize for differences in the age and sex distribution of the groups under comparison.[80]

Preventive Services Consistent racial differences exist in preventive care in children. For example, fewer white children (9 percent) than non-white children (15 percent) have never had a physical examination.[81] Poorer preventive care among non-white children is also evident in data (displayed in Table 3) on immunizations against infectious diseases. These data, compiled by the Center for Disease Control (CDC), show that the immunization rate for white children is consistently higher than the rate for children from "other races." On the other hand, a 1976 national survey conducted by the Center for Health Administration Studies found no racial differences in polio, measles, and DPT vaccinations, as reported by parents.[82] (Because this survey shows much higher percentages of children to be vaccinated than did the CDC study, there is a possibility that parents overreport the vaccination of their children.)

There is some evidence of similar deficits in preventive care among Hispanic populations. In the mid-1970s, large surveys in Alameda County, California, found that although Mexican Americans reported the same number of physician visits as English-speaking whites the former were less likely to report having had a general examination or eye examinations either in the past year or ever.[83] These differences persisted, though at a reduced level, even after statistical controls for the effects of education and family income.

Racial Differences in Source of Ambulatory Care Virtually the same proportions of the black (86.3 percent) and white (87.7 percent) populations reported in the 1978 Health Interview Survey that they

Table 3. PERCENTAGE OF CHILDREN IMMUNIZED AGAINST FIVE INFECTIOUS DISEASES, BY RACE, 1978

	Rubella[1]	Measles[1]	3+ Doses DPT[2]	3+ Doses Polio[2]	3+ Doses Mumps[1]
White	69	73	74	69	55
Non-white	57	58	56	49	46

[1]Includes ages 1-14.
[2]Includes ages 0-14.

SOURCE: Center for Disease Control, U.S. Immmunization Survey: 1978.

have a "usual source of care." (Among those who do not have a usual source of care, whites are much more likely than non-whites to report that they previously have had a regular source of care.[84]) However, there are striking racial differences in where care is obtained. Roberts and Lee found a similar pattern among blacks, whites, and Chicanos in Alameda County; although there was little difference in having a regular source of care or in physician visits, there were notable differences in the source of medical care.[85]

Such patterns are evident in national data from the Health Interview Survey (Table 4). The first two columns show that, although there is little racial difference in having a usual source of medical care, whites are somewhat more likely than blacks to report that they usually see one particular doctor. Whites are much more likely than blacks to report their usual source of care to be an office-based physician and less likely to report outpatient departments and health centers as their usual source of care. Table 4 also shows that, while both types of insurance (private and Medicare vs. Medicaid) and income level affect people's usual source of medical care, a racial difference persists even within different income groups and among people who have similar types of health insurance. Thus, it is clear that more than poverty underlies the racial disparities in where people obtain their medical care.

Racial differences in the source of care also are evident in a community study of the health care of rural and "urban fringe" blacks and whites in North Carolina, where "74 percent of the rural and 64 percent of the urban whites named a private physician as their usual source of care, against 22 and 18 percent of blacks in the respective areas."[86] The researchers concluded that, because so few blacks and Medicaid patients were served by community physicians (and thus served by neighborhood health centers and county health departments), "removal of legal and financial barriers has made little impact as yet on the patterns of health care delivery established before the institution of mandatory integration of health services."[87]

Table 4. USUAL SOURCE OF MEDICAL CARE, BY RACE, INSURANCE, AND INCOME LEVEL, 1978 (Percentages)

	Total		Type of Insurance						Income Level			
			Private Insurance/ Medicare		Medicaid Only		None		Less Than 150% of Poverty Level		More Than Twice the Poverty Level	
	White	Black	White	Black	White	Black	White	Black	White	Black	White	Black
Has A Usual Source of Medical Care	88	86	89	87	90	92	77	79	86	88	88	83
Usually Sees One Particular Doctor	74	60	76	66	67	53	62	46	69	56	75	62
What is Usual Source of Care?												
Office-Based Physician	77	58	79	65	67	46	63	44	70	52	78	59
Out-Patient Department	4	13	3	10	10	22	5	15	6	18	4	11
Emergency Room	1	3	1	2	2	3	1	6	1	4	1	3
Health Center	1	6	1	4	6	14	3	8	3	9	1	4

SOURCE: National Center for Health Statistics. Health Interview Survey, 1978. Unpublished data.

A second type of racial disparity in people's sources of medical care concerns the use of medical specialists. Table 5 shows the way in which physician visits by blacks and whites are distributed across physician specialties, as reported in household interviews. The table shows that a slightly greater percentage of physician visits by black patients than of white patients are to general practitioners.

When the major settings for physician visits are examined, much larger racial differences appear. Table 6 shows the racial distribution of physician contacts by specialty, according to whether they took place in the office of a private physician, in a hospital clinic or emergency room, or over the telephone. (The small number of physician visits at other sites--at home or at work, for example--are not included in this table.) Physician contacts by telephone were more than twice as common for whites as for blacks. In addition, physician visits for blacks were twice as likely as for whites to take place in hospital clinics and emergency rooms; visits with internists and pediatricians were more than three times as likely for blacks as for whites to take place in such settings. This suggests that private practitioners are more available to whites than to blacks. Although there is evidence that some organized health care settings can provide good-quality care to poverty patients,[88] a large literature suggests that the use of hospital clinics and emergency rooms as a usual source of care has serious deficiencies. Nevertheless, little evidence exists that allows systematic comparison of quality of medical care across the types of sites discussed herein.

Associated with the racial differences in sources of care are differences in the ease with which people obtain care. "Difficulty getting to the doctor" was second only to cost as a barrier to care cited by poor people and non-whites questioned in the 1974 Health Interview Survey,[89] and surveys such as those conducted by the National Center for Health Statistics (NCHS) and the Center for Health Administration Studies (CHAS) have consistently found that the travel time of non-whites exceeds that of whites. For example, 1976 CHAS data show 49 percent of whites and 40 percent of non-whites travel less than 15 minutes to reach their usual source of care.[90] How much of the racial difference in travel time is due to differences in the distance traveled, and how much is due to differences in modes of transportation, cannot be ascertained directly from the available data. However, in the CHAS data, the racial difference was present, though reduced, within income categories.[91] NCHS data, presented in Table 7, show that black travel time exceeds white travel time no matter what income or type of insurance they have. The same unpublished data from the 1978 Health Interview Survey also show racial differences in travel time among persons who live in metropolitan areas (data not shown), notwithstanding the greater use by poor blacks of what might seem to be "local" sources of care--neighborhood health centers and hospital clinics and emergency rooms.

Explanations of Racial/Ethnic Patterns in Ambulatory Care Data presented thus far show that (1) although some racial/ethnic differences in receipt of medical care have disappeared, minority groups, taken as a whole, remain at a disadvantage by some measures; (2) consistent racial/ethnic differences remain in the sources from which people obtain medical care;

Table 5. PERCENTAGE OF PHYSICIAN VISITS, BY RACE OF PATIENT AND SPECIALTY OF PHYSICIAN, 1978

Specialty of Physician	Race of Patient	
	White	Black
General Practitioner	48.5	54.6
Dermatologist	1.7	1.5
Internist	10.5	5.5
OB, GYN	6.8	6.5
Ophthalmologist	2.5	1.5
Orthopedist	4.3	2.4
Otolaryngologist	2.3	1.3
Pediatrician	9.5	8.2
Psychiatrist	1.1	1.0
Radiologist	1.2	0.6
Surgeon	3.0	2.7
Urologist	1.3	2.0
Other Specialists	3.2	5.3
Unknown	3.6	6.5
Total	100.0%	100.0%

SOURCE: National Center for Health Statistics. 1978 Health Interview Survey, unpublished data.

and (3) whites seeking medical care use less travel time, on average, than do blacks. A number of factors may possibly explain at least part of these differences. These include racial/ethnic differences in preferences for various sources of care, racial/ethnic differences in ability to pay for medical care, spatial patterns in the location of populations and sources of medical care, and discrimination by providers either against minority group members or against classes (for example, Medicaid patients) of which some minority groups constitute a disproportionate share.

Literature in the social sciences shows that differences in values affect virtually every kind of human behavior, including seeking medical care. However, although different values and other cultural factors undoubtedly influence whether people seek medical attention when particular symptoms are experienced, it seems unlikely that minority groups' disproportionate use of clinics and emergency rooms and their expenditure of greater amounts of travel time to obtain care are to an important degree a true expression of preferences. Not only is there little evidence to suggest this is true, but competing explanations are more plausible.

A set of factors that undoubtedly affects patterns of medical care relates to cost. Disproportionate numbers of both black and Hispanic populations in the United States are found in low-income

Table 6. PERCENT DISTRIBUTION OF PLACE OF PHYSICIAN VISITS, BY PHYSICIAN SPECIALTY AND RACE OF PATIENT, 1978

		Place of Visit			
Physician Specialty	Race of Patient	Physician's Office	Hospital Clinic/ Emergency Room	Tele-phone	Total[1]
General	White	70	11	13	100%
Practitioner	Black	60	24	4	100%
Internist	White	70	10	15	100%
	Black	55	33	*	100%
OB, GYN	White	76	8	13	100%
	Black	68	13	12	100%
Pediatrician	White	69	5	25	100%
	Black	56	18	20	100%
Total[2]	White	69	12	13	100%
	Black	57	25	5	100%

*Too few cases for reliable percentage to be calculated.
[1]Rows add to less than 100 percent because some visit sites are not shown and because of missing data.
[2]Table includes only specialties with sufficient numbers to allow for calculation of percentage distributions across visit sites. The total rows, however, include all physician visits.

SOURCE: National Center for Health Statistics. 1978 Health Interview Survey, unpublished data.

categories.[92] Furthermore, disproportionate numbers of the poor have no insurance coverage for medical care; this is particularly true for the Mexican-American population of the Southwest.[93] Considerable evidence exists that ability to pay (including having insurance) has marked effects on people's ability to obtain health care.[94] In addition, because of the association between racial/ethnic status and poverty, the Medicaid rolls include disproportionate numbers of minority persons. Yet it is also clear that these factors do not suffice as an explanation of racial/ethnic differences in medical care, because, as has already been noted, substantial racial/ethnic differences exist within income and insurance categories.

Nevertheless, there can be no doubt that differences in income and in Medicaid status influence the racial/ethnic patterns that have been described in this chapter. This is particularly obvious in the case of income, because under the present health care system in the United States only a limited number of public facilities are available to provide care to persons unable to pay for it. The health care system is designed to concentrate persons who cannot pay in a few

Table 7. PERCENT TRAVELING MORE THAN 29 MINUTES TO USUAL SOURCE OF MEDICAL CARE, 1978

	White	Black
Type of Insurance		
Private Insurance and Medicare	15.0	18.6
Medicaid Only	20.5	25.3
None	15.4	23.8
Income Level		
More than Twice Poverty Level	16.2	19.2
Less than 150% of Poverty Level	20.0	23.8
Total	15.4	20.8

SOURCE: National Center for Health Statistics. 1978 Health Interview Survey, unpublished tables.

facilities. (The so-called "free care" provisions of the Hill-Burton Act, described in Chapter 5, have had little effect on this because they have not been enforced and because hospitals see obvious economic disadvantages in providing care to people who cannot pay for it.) The increasingly common accounts of poor patients (including Medicaid patients in some cities) being "dumped" from the emergency rooms of voluntary or private hospitals into public hospitals (with grave economic consequences for the latter) is one example of the pervasive phenomenon of each element in the health care system (including both providers and different levels of government) seeking to shift costs elsewhere. One consequence of this trend is almost certainly the concentration of poor and minority patients into relatively few, economically unhealthy facilities.

Spatial Distribution of Medical Resources Many studies have shown that the spatial distribution of health manpower does not mirror the distribution of the U.S. population.[95] Most of these studies have focused on rural-urban differences and have called attention to the manpower problems of rural parts of the United States. However, because the minority population of the United States is disproportionately urban, these studies are of limited usefulness in explaining the racial patterns that have been outlined in this chapter. More useful are the studies that have been conducted at the local level.

The relative scarcity of private physicians in urban neighborhoods in which ethnic minorities predominate has been documented in a variety of studies. Most of this research involves analyses of the relationship between the supply of physicians in different areas (such as census tracts) of a city and certain characteristics of the areas--median income, mean age, availability of hospital beds, and so forth. Most of this research is directed at understanding patterns of physician location, and it is concerned less with describing the resources available to minority communities than with considering the racial or ethnic characteristics of an area as one of many factors that may "explain" physician-location patterns.

These studies show that physicians' offices tend not to be located in areas where there is a predominance of black and Hispanic residents.[96] Such research in some cities has found that the racial factor operates independently of the other factors studied (median income, supply of hospital beds, and so forth),[97] although there are also indications that in more middle-class black communities the problem is much less pronounced, in part, because of the locational preferences of black physicians.[98]

Whatever the relative importance of class and racial factors, it is clear that the overwhelming burden of social-class differentials with regard to proximity to physician services falls on non-whites. This is seen both through correlational studies regarding the relationship between physician supply and race of residents[99] and descriptive studies of the characteristics of poor, minority neighborhoods. Thus, several of the poorest neighborhoods in New York City are reported as having as few as 0.15 office-based physicians for every 1,000 residents.[100] Evidence from a Chicago study showed the concentration of physicians in affluent neighborhoods to have increased between 1950 and 1970; the 10 most affluent communities saw their physician/population ratio rise from 1.78 to 2.1/1,000 in that period; within the 10 poorest communities, the ratio dropped from 0.99 to 0.26/1,000.[101]

Although the scarcity of private physicians is an important fact of life in neighborhoods occupied by minorities and the poor, it does not suffice as an explanation of racial differences in the source of health care. Regarding use of hospitals, several studies (reviewed later in this chapter) show that travel beyond the nearest facility seems to be a common pattern among urban blacks. Similar patterns exist with regard to ambulatory care. Data from a 1968-71 survey conducted in 10 cities shows that, even within the same general neighborhoods, large racial differences exist in where people obtain medical care, as is shown in Table 8.[102] The data strongly suggest that the disproportionate use by blacks of hospitals and public clinics cannot be attributed simply to proximity, because the usual source of medical care for whites in the same neighborhoods consistently differs from that of blacks. These differences were very large in some cases; in southeast Philadelphia, for example, more than half of blacks, but fewer than 10 percent of whites, reported that a hospital or public clinic was their usual source of medical care. Furthermore, Table 8 also shows that the travel time of blacks to their medical care is consistently larger than whites who reside in the same general area of the city. (Whether this reflects a difference in mode of transportation or in distance traveled is again not clear.) The important point is that factors other than the geographic distribution of medical resources affect racial differences in where people obtain medical care. For some reason, blacks in these areas make less use of private physicians than do whites.

Table 8. USUAL SOURCE OF CARE AND TRAVEL TIME AMONG RESIDENTS OF 10 URBAN AREAS, BY RACE, 1968-71

Area and Survey Year	Percent Reporting Hospitals and Public Clinics as Usual Source of Care		Percent Traveling 30 Minutes or More to Usual Source of Care	
	Black	White	Black	White
Roxbury, Boston, MA. 1971	76	59	60	52
Bedford Stuyvesant-Crown Heights, Brooklyn. 1968	43	14	58	40
Red Hook, Brooklyn. 1968-69	30	6	52	38
Southeast Philadelphia, PA. 1968-69	53	9	44	35
Upper Cardozo, Washington, D.C. 1969	40	18	60	59
Southside, Atlanta, GA. 1968	72	21	78	58
Peninsula, Charleston, SC. 1969	56	11	51	21
Wayne Minor & Model Cities Area. Kansas City, MO. 1969-70	51	36	60	51
Mission, San Francisco, CA. 1970	31	17	66	65
East Palo Alto, CA. 1969	12	8	28	26

SOURCE: Louise M. Okada and Gerald Sparer, "Access to Usual Source of Care by Race and Income in Ten Urban Areas," Journal of Community Health 1 (Spring 1976) pp. 163-174.

Discrimination by Physicians Many of the data presented thus far--most notably the findings that blacks make less use of private physicians than do whites with similar incomes and insurance coverage and that black and white residents of the same general urban areas use different sources of care--are consistent with the hypothesis that minority group use of health care is influenced by patterns of discrimination among physicians. Despite scattered reports of physician discrimination in the form of segregated waiting rooms or office hours,[103] no data exist on the extent to which racial discrimination exists in actually accepting patients for treatment. That a hospital that excluded black patients could still exist in the late 1970s lends plausibility to the possibility that some individual practitioners may still practice discrimination.[104]

It was initially hoped that the Medicaid program might help integrate eligible persons into the mainstream health care delivery system. Its success in doing so depends in substantial part on an adequate level of participation by providers. For various reasons, including low payment levels, a significant proportion of physicians apparently do not accept Medicaid patients, although the existing estimates of physician participation are very imprecise. In a national survey of more than 3,300 physicians conducted by the National Opinion Research Corporation in 1975-76, 77 percent of responding physicians answered affirmatively to the question "Do you participate in your state's Medicaid program; that is, do you receive payment from Medicaid?"[105] This figure should be interpreted carefully, however, for three reasons. First, not all specialties were included (although the most common ones were), and because members of minorities are found in disproportionately small numbers in specialists' practices, leaving out some specialties may artificially inflate the estimate of the percentage that accepts Medicaid patients. Second, one-third of the physicians did not return their questionnaire; although the authors show that these non-respondents were similar to respondents in some regards, the possibility exists that they were different with regard to acceptance of Medicaid patients. Third, physicians who had as few as one Medicaid patient may have answered affirmatively to the question regarding acceptance of Medicaid. Thus, Mitchell and Cromwell also examined Medicaid patients as a percentage of physicians' practices, and found that, in addition to the 23 percent of physicians who had no Medicaid patients, another 27 percent had fewer than 10 percent Medicaid patients.[106]

Perhaps the best indicator of the availability of physicians to Medicaid patients is whether they would accept new Medicaid patients. A survey of general practitioners conducted by Mathematica Policy Research in 1975 showed as many as half were not taking new Medicaid patients, as is shown in Table 9. These rates are for general practitioners, and it is probable that they overestimate overall physician acceptance of Medicaid patients, because Medicaid participation in many specialties is much lower.[107] Physician acceptance of Medicaid patients was particularly low in the South and in large cities, which coincides with the location of the bulk of minority group members in the United States. Table 9 also includes, for comparison purposes, figures on physician participation in Medicare. Physician participation is consistently higher in Medicare than in Medicaid, which may be due to the size of the market (there are more Medicare patients than Medicaid patients, and they use more care) and to higher rates of reimbursement.[108] However, the data are also consistent with the hypothesis of racial discrimination. Differences in physician acceptance of Medicare and Medicaid patients are most pronounced in areas where racial/ethnic minority groups are concentrated. Thus, in the non-metropolitan Northeast and West, only

Table 9. GENERAL PRACTITIONERS' ACCEPTANCE OF MEDICARE AND MEDICAID PATIENTS, BY AREA AND REGION, 1975

Region	Percent Patients Medicare	Percent Taking New Medicare Patients	Percent Patients Medicaid	Percent Taking New Medicaid Patients
Large SMSAs				
Northeast	25.9	79.9	12.4	56.2
North Central	25.6	78.3	12.9	52.1
South	27.3	78.3	10.9	42.8
West	29.3	84.5	17.0	49.9
Small SMSAs				
Northeast	30.3	84.8	19.8	73.0
North Central	26.3	80.3	12.9	53.7
South	26.0	67.5	15.8	46.0
West	21.8	83.3	17.9	61.6
Non-metropolitan				
Northeast	36.1	85.0	19.7	78.5
North Central	28.0	75.9	12.4	65.0
South	25.3	60.6	18.8	51.3
West	19.8	64.6	13.5	58.7
Totals				
Large SMSAs	26.9	79.8	12.9	49.7
Small SMSAs	26.1	76.3	16.2	55.2
Non-metropolitan	26.8	68.8	16.4	59.9

SOURCE: The Physician Capacity Utilization Surveys: Special Analyses, DHEW Publication No. (HRA) 79-30, (Washington, D.C.: DHEW, 1979) p. 225.

about 7 percent more physicians accept new Medicare patients than Medicaid patients. On the other hand, more than one-third more physicians in large cities of the South and West will accept new Medicare patients than will accept new Medicaid patients. (The non-metropolitan South, it should be noted, is not notably different from other non-metropolitan areas of the country regarding the difference in acceptance of new Medicare and Medicaid patients.)

Quality of Ambulatory Care In discussing the results of a study they conducted in the rural South in the mid-1970s, Davis and Marshall make the following observations about what they learned about racial differences in the quality of medical care:

> Cursory, inadequate physical examinations are frequently given to minority patients. In some places, rural blacks are unaware that it is customary to undress for medical examinations while this procedure is common among whites in the same area. Blood pressure readings are taken through the clothing of black patients, thus increasing the risk of inadequate measurements, a particularly serious problem for blacks with a high incidence of hypertension. Minority women are less likely to receive professional preventive services such as Pap smears and breast examinations. High rates of hysterectomies are also seen in some areas.[109]

Unfortunately, no description has been published of the methods used in this study, and no data are presented on the frequency of these shortcomings in the medical care of blacks and whites. However, echoes of these findings can be heard in Senator Moss's account of three "Medicaid mills" that he visited in New York City while posing as a patient. Moss writes of dirty facilities, impersonal care, unnecessary tests and prescriptions, and blood pressure and pulse readings being taken through clothing.[110] It is difficult to define the role played by the racial/ethnic characteristics of patients in the patterns of care that Davis and Marshall and Moss describe. However, when such accounts are considered in light of the history of racial discrimination in the United States, the association between race/ethnicity and income, and the segregated patterns described earlier in this chapter, it is reasonable to ask whether there are racial differences in the quality of medical care provided.

Great interest has arisen about the quality of medical care, and an active research literature has developed.[111] This literature, which suggests that important deficiencies occur in the medical care of Americans, provides relatively little systematic information about racial differences in the quality of medical care.[112] Indications that a racial difference exists in the quality of care is provided by some of the information already presented in this chapter; however, more direct measures are also available.

One determinant of quality of medical care is the competence of the physician providing care. A number of studies have shown that the quality of care in a medical setting is influenced by factors such as the percentage of specialists practicing there and the length of their training.[113] As was noted earlier in this chapter, more of the care provided to minority groups than to whites is provided by non-specialists. Furthermore, there are indications that less than fully qualified foreign medical graduates provide care in state-financed medical institutions, particularly state mental hospitals, where the patients are disproportionately poor and black.[114]

Studies of physicians providing care to Medicaid patients provides some useful, inferential material about the care of poor members of minority groups, although many Medicaid patients are not from minority groups. Relatively few physicians provide care to relatively large numbers of Medicaid patients; estimates from a national survey suggest that 5 percent of the physicians in the country may provide care to one-third of the Medicaid patients.[115] Physicians who provide care to relatively large numbers of Medicaid patients include disproportionate numbers of general practitioners, and, because of the negative association between age and specialty training, they tend to be older than the average physician.[116] Foreign medical graduates also provide a disproportionate amount of the care to Medicaid patients.[117] Kavaler's study of 126 physicians participating in the Medicaid program in the black and Puerto Rican slums of New York City found that 35 percent had no access to hospital beds and 42 percent had only limited privileges at proprietary hospitals.[118] (Alers also reviews data that raises questions about the qualifications of some physicians providing care in Puerto Rican neighborhoods in New York.)[119] Similar results were reported from a study in Chicago.[120] Because of such characteristics of physicians who treat relatively large numbers of Medicaid patients, Mitchell and Cromwell suggest that the Medicaid program and its beneficiaries constitute a "secondary, residual market" for medical care.[121] That is, the physicians least able to compete in the medical market--because of foreign training, lack of specialty credentials, or lack of hospital privileges--end up providing much of the care for Medicaid patients. Thus, "a primary goal of the public benefits programs to integrate the poor into mainstream medicine is thereby thwarted."[122]

Patient satisfaction provides another aspect of possible differences in the quality of medical care. Patients' assessments of the care they receive are influenced by a variety of factors, including waiting time and time spent with physicians,[123] and cannot be considered a measure of quality in a strict medical sense. Nevertheless, patients are the only persons who are in a position to judge certain aspects of the care that they receive, and their perceptions of that care should be taken seriously.

The best available evidence shows higher levels of dissatisfaction with various aspects of medical care among both blacks and Hispanics than among whites. Table 10 shows such racial/ethnic (as well as income) differences in patients' evaluations of several aspects of the care that they receive--its convenience and availability, the financing of care, the humaneness of doctors, the quality of care, and

Table 10. PERCENT MORE DISSATISFIED THAN THE MEDIAN PERSON WITH ASPECTS OF MEDICAL CARE, BY RACE AND POVERTY LEVEL, 1976[1]

	Percent More Dissatisfied Than Median						
Race and Poverty Level	Convenience of Services	Availability of Services	Financing of Care	Humaneness of Doctors	Quality of Care	General Dissatisfaction	
White	48	48	49	50	50	48	(4,332)[2]
Spanish heritage, Southwest	54	50	59	45	49	55	(616)
Above poverty level	55	45	65	46	46	55	(343)
Below poverty level	54	56	51	43	51	56	(273)
Other white	48	48	49	50	50	48	(3,716)
Above poverty level	45	45	47	50	49	46	(3,087)
Below poverty level	62	59	59	53	57	55	(629)
Non-white	67	71	54	55	52	64	(803)
Non-SMSA black, South	76	86	62	59	56	68	(399)
Above poverty level	72	86	66	60	58	67	(164)
Below poverty level	79	86	59	58	56	68	(235)
Other non-white	65	67	52	54	51	63	(404)
Above poverty level	63	68	54	51	49	62	(265)
Below poverty level	69	64	49	59	55	65	(139)
Total	50	50	50	50	50	50	(5,135)

[1]Percent table N is of U.S. adult population equals 95; percent NA equals 5.
[2]In parentheses are the unweighted numbers of observations. Since the 1976 sample is a weighted sample, these numbers should not be used for combining subcategories.

SOURCE: Lu Ann Aday, Ronald Andersen, and Gretchen V. Fleming, Health Care in the U.S.: Equitable for Whom? (Beverly Hills, CA: Sage, 1980) p. 153.

overall dissatisfaction. The data, taken from the most recent national survey conducted by the Center for Health Administration Studies, show generally higher levels of dissatisfaction among both the "Spanish heritage, Southwest" sample and among blacks than among whites, and appear to reflect, at least in part, differences in the source of care.[124] The racial/ethnic differences were generally more pronounced on the measures of convenience and availability than on the measures of performance of physicians (humaneness and quality), although that has not been found in all studies.[125] A majority of persons expressed satisfaction with the various dimensions of medical care,[126] and although perceptions of the same objective reality may differ, the pattern seems clear that whites are more satisfied with their medical care than are blacks and the Hispanic population of the Southwest.

Hospital Care

The most recent national surveys do not show consistent or striking differences among whites, blacks, and Hispanics in the rate of hospitalization.[127] However, this may not indicate that blacks and whites have the same access to hospital care when it is needed. Since a variety of serious health problems are more common among blacks than among whites, equivalent access to care might be expected to produce higher rates of hospitalization among blacks. (Indeed, data for enlisted Naval personnel, whose access to care is presumably only minimally affected by race, show higher rates of hospitalization for blacks than for whites.[128])

Data from both the Health Interview Survey and the Hospital Discharge Survey show the length of stay for blacks to be higher than for whites.[129] Whether this indicates a racial difference in patients' condition upon admission, as is sometimes suggested, is speculative.

There are some indications that hospitalized blacks are slightly less likely than whites to have surgery,[130] although assessment of the meaning of this difference is most uncertain. Hospital Discharge Survey data also show great variation in the ratio of whites to non-whites in the incidence of different surgical procedures.[131] However, given both the level of aggregation in the published data and the amount of missing racial data in the Hospital Discharge Survey, no conclusions can be drawn about racial trends.

Regarding a set of surgical procedures about which particular concern has been expressed over the years--sterilization--available data show earlier racial differences in incidence to have largely disappeared. Data from the Hospital Discharge Survey, for example, show that, in 1971, black women were undergoing tubal sterilization at a rate of 12 per 1,000 women aged 15-44, while the comparable rate for white women was 5.3; by 1975, the rate of tubal sterilization among blacks was still 12 per 1,000, while the rate for whites was 11.6 per 1,000.[132] Similar trends are evident in survey data published by the National Center for Health Statistics. As of 1976, among women aged 15-45 who had ever been married, blacks (13.1 percent) were more likely than whites (10.5 percent) and Hispanics (9.4 percent) to have ever undergone a tubal ligation.*[133] However, in the years between 1973 and 1976, the incidence of tubal ligation was slightly higher among whites (5.7 percent) than among blacks (5.5 percent) or Hispanics (4.7 percent). Data on hysterectomies showed little difference between blacks and whites in ever having the surgery (approximately 8 percent of both groups) or having had it in the previous three years (approximately 4 percent of both groups). The rate of hysterectomies among Hispanic women aged 15-45 was somewhat lower.

The topic of sterilization of minority groups has also been linked to concerns about informed consent for several years, having received considerable attention in Senate hearings held in 1973.[135] Following those hearings, regulatory changes were made in Medicaid that attempted to set conditions more conducive to informed consent and to limit the use of hysterectomy for sterilization purposes. No systematic studies of the effects of those regulations have been published. However, there is an imperfect indicator of racial differences in the incidence of sterilization under conditions that may be questionable from the standpoint of informed consent: the percentage of tubal ligations performed on women who were pregnant when hospitalized. Because the hospitalization is for a purpose other than sterilization, the possibility is increased that the woman might not understand that a sterilization procedure is involved. Informed consent procedures undertaken as part of the process of labor and childbirth can easily go awry.[136] Therefore, consent is better obtained prior to hospitalization. Although no data are available regarding when consent is obtained for sterilization, both the regulations and the concern about the issue may have been responsible for a large decrease between 1970 and 1975 in the proportion of tubal ligations performed on women who were pregnant when hospitalized. However, in the most recent year for which data are available (1975), 59.7 percent of the black women who underwent tubal ligation were pregnant when hospitalized, compared with 41.5 percent of white women. While this difference may be a reflection of racial differences in fertility,[137] it points to a potential source of consent problems that is more common among blacks than among whites.

<u>Patterns of Hospital Use</u> The racial patterns in physician visits have parallels in patterns of hospitalization, although no national data exist that are comparable to the data reviewed above on racial

*When this report was written, all available data from the NCHS interview survey were for women who had been married. However, never married women make up a significant proportion (22.1 percent) of black women who underwent tubal sterilization in 1975, compared with only 2.3 percent of white women.[134] Thus, data that are limited to the incidence of sterilization among ever married women may possibly obscure continuing racial differences.

patterns in the use of physicians. Studies conducted in several cities, however, describe the elements of a dual track system. This is true of all cities for which information is available on racial patterns in hospital care.

Comprehensive studies of the workings of entire urban medical care systems are scarce. One of the best studies was of Chicago over a 15-year period ending in 1965. It found that blacks were hospitalized in a very small subset of the more than 150 hospitals in the metropolitan area.[138] Fifty percent of all black patients in Chicago traveled to one hospital, Cook County General Hospital, where 85 percent of the patients were black.[139] Another 30 percent of black patients were served by five university-affiliated teaching hospitals and one (of three) traditionally "black" hospital. Writing in the late 1960s, DeVise described the racial trends in hospitalization as follows:

> The dual system of Negro indigent patient hospitals and white private patient hospitals has persisted even though extensive Medicare and Medicaid programs now reimburse private hospitals and physicians for the care of indigents; even though OEO and Children's Bureau now pay private hospitals to set up free neighborhood health centers and pediatric clinics; even though there has been a sevenfold increase in the number of Negro physicians admitted to practice in private white hospitals; even though the Negro ghetto has more than doubled in area, absorbing in the process six more white hospitals; even though the average distance from Negro homes to Cook County Hospital has increased from five to eight miles, while the average distance from Negro homes to white hospitals stayed under one mile.[140]

A vivid measure of the nature of the travel patterns involved in the use of Cook County Hospital comes from the calculation that the 500,000 patient miles per month that were traveled to Cook County Hospital would be reduced to 50,000 miles if patients used the hospital nearest their homes.[141] The average distance traveled by all black patients to the various Chicago hospitals where they were admitted was six miles; the average trip for a white patient was three miles.[142]

Travel time was also used as an indicator of a racial dual track system in a study of hospital use in Cleveland.[143] Seventy-four percent of the blacks surveyed, compared with 59 percent of whites, traveled beyond the hospital that was second nearest to their home. The authors noted that personal and cultural preferences can lead to travel to a hospital. Thus, for example, Jews were particularly likely to travel beyond the second nearest hospital (92 percent did so) in order to make use of one particular hospital--Mt. Sinai. The authors noted, however, that "the concentration of blacks at Metropolitan General Hospital suggests a different set of constraints featuring poverty and discrimination."[144]

Descriptive material on racial patterns in hospitalization are also available for New Orleans, where data were assembled in connection with a race discrimination suit (Cook v. Ochsner Foundation Hospital, et al.) brought by the Department of Health, Education, and Welfare in 1970. These data, which are included in a summary of the Cook case that is presented in Appendix E of this report, showed blacks to be concentrated in two hospitals; of blacks that had been hospitalized in 1974-77, 75 percent had gone to 2 of the 16 hospitals in metropolitan New Orleans.[145] Conversely, blacks were underrepresented in other New Orleans hospitals.

Identifiably "black" hospitals and associated patterns of racial segregation continue to exist to some degree in hospitals in many other cities, although no systematic analysis has been done on the topic. However, applicable research methodologies have been developed in studies of segregation in other areas, such as education and residence,[146] and data that are potentially useful for describing racial patterns of where people obtain medical care exist from programs such as Medicare and Medicaid. In principle, studies could be done of the degree of segregation in hospital use in various cities, the extent of its variation from city to city, and whether it is increasing or decreasing in response to factors such as economic trends and civil rights enforcement activity.

Quality of Care in Hospitals Existing studies of quality have generally not examined racial and ethnic issues. Nevertheless, despite the complexities of defining and measuring quality, several existing approaches can be used to detect at least gross disparities that may deserve closer examination. These approaches include studies of resources (especially personnel), treatment processes, and outcomes.

Within medical institutions, there are indications that care is provided to minority groups by less well trained physicians. Studies of this matter are not common, perhaps because of its sensitivity. Duff and Hollingshead showed that the social class of patients had a pervasive impact on their care at a large university hospital.[147] The class position of patients, for example, influenced whether a patient was managed by a "committee," with no one clearly identifiable to the patient as responsible for his or her case, or whether the patient had a "committed" sponsor in the hospital. Although this study provided extensive documentation of the effects of class in hospital care, it was confined to whites.

More direct evidence about the racial factor in hospitals comes from Egbert and Rothman's study of the relationship between patient characteristics and the training of their surgeon at a teaching hospital.[148] Blacks were much more likely than whites to be under the care of surgeons in training (that is, a resident surgeon) rather than a staff physician. For example, among patients who were "paying directly or with commercial insurance," 34 percent of blacks and 7 percent of whites were treated by a resident surgeon. However, among Medicaid patients, no statistically significant racial difference was found; more than 40 percent of both white and black Medicaid patients were treated by residents. Egbert and Rothman also found that among emergency patients, blacks were twice as likely as whites to be treated by a resident. Egbert and Rothman's study was based on medical records and could easily be duplicated at other institutions and for other types of care. However, no other well-documented accounts appear in the literature in which racial differences within institutions are examined.

Similar racial/ethnic sorting processes have been described in mental health settings. For example, Flaherty and Meagher, in a study of 66 black and 36 white male schizophrenic inpatients, found blacks to be more likely than whites to have been given medications on an "as needed" basis, less likely to have received recreation therapy and occupational therapy, and more likely to have been put in seclusion and to have had restraints used.[149] These differences appeared to have been due to subtle racial stereotyping among staff members and their greater familiarity with white patients, rather than to racial differences in pathology. In a study of racial differences in the treatment of children in five mental health clinics, Jackson, Berkowitz, and Farley found that black children were less likely than white children to be accepted for treatment, less likely to receive individual treatment, and (at two clinics) to be seen for a lesser length of time.[150]

In his study of services provided to members of different ethnic groups in 17 centers in Seattle, Sue found significant differences in the types of personnel seen both at intake and during therapy.[151] At intake and during therapy, blacks saw significantly fewer psychiatrists, psychololgists, social workers, and nurses, and more "other professionals," non-professionals, and "other personnel," than did whites.[152] This was true even after demographic differences were controlled statistically. However, no consistent pattern of differences from whites were found among the ethnic groups studied. Thus, for example, American Indians saw more social workers and fewer non-professionals than did whites, Asian Americans saw fewer professionals than did whites, and Chicanos did not differ significantly from whites in the kind of personnel seen. Sue also examined ethnic differences in diagnoses, the type of program and the number of sessions in which patients became involved, and their rates of premature dropping out (an indicator of the effectiveness of the program). All of the results are summarized in Table 11, which shows different patterns of treatment among the different ethnic groups, with blacks differing from whites on all the variables examined. When statistical controls were introduced to eliminate the effects of ethnic differences in age, sex, education, income, and marital status, members of all of the ethnic groups were still significantly more likely than whites to terminate prematurely their course of treatment.

Over the years, the psychiatric literature has shown more evidence of concern about possible racial bias in treatment than has the literature of any other area of health care. Considerable evidence exists of serious concern about racism and mental health. The problem of cultural differences is a particularly difficult one in the field of mental health because of the nature of both the problems that are addressed and the theoretical conceptions that have been

Table 11. SUMMARY OF FINDINGS REGARDING ETHNIC-WHITE DIFFERENCES IN PATIENTS AT 17 COMMUNITY MENTAL HEALTH FACILITIES

	Blacks	Native Americans	Asian Americans	Chicanos
Utilization Rates	+	+	-	-
No. of Demographic Differences	5	3	3	3
Significant Diagnosis Differences	Yes	No	No	No
Type Staff Seen at Intake	Yes	Yes	Yes	No
Type Staff Seen in Therapy	Yes	No	Yes	No
Type of Program	Yes	No	No	No
Type of Service	Yes	No	No	No
Number of Sessions	Yes	Yes	Yes	Yes
Premature Termination	Yes	Yes	Yes	Yes

SOURCE: Stanley Sue, "Community Mental Health Services to Minority Groups: Some Optimism, Some Pessimism," American Psychologist (August 1977), pp. 616-624.

dominant. These problems have not been addressed in detail in this report and perhaps cannot be examined within the broad focus that it takes. That serious efforts have been made within the field to assess the operation of racial/ethnic biases in treatment is evidence of concern about these problems. The results of this research suggest that concern by those outside the field is also warranted.

Another approach makes use of existing information to examine differences in the process by which care is provided. An example is Shaw's study using 1968 hospital discharge information from the Commission on Professional and Hospital Activities.[153] He found differences between whites and blacks in the rates that various diagnostic and therapeutic techniques were documented in medical records, as is shown in Table 12. Furthermore, the data show that these racial differences were less likely to occur in small hospitals than in large hospitals, and were less likely to occur in the western section of the United States than in the remainder of the country.

The presentation of Shaw's data does not allow judgments to be made regarding inequities in medical care. The operational details used were not described, and the nature of the racial differences was not indicated. Nevertheless, the methodology itself appears to be powerful and worth pursuing, at least in an exploratory or research mode. Its potential for better documenting differences in care, many of which have strong quality implications, appears promising.

Studies of Outcomes of Hospital Care Differences in treatment cause concern, at least in part, because of suspicions that such will produce differences in the health of people. However, researchers have found it difficult to link process and outcome measures of quality of care. Although differences in process are of themselves

Table 12. LIST OF STATISTICALLY SIGNIFICANT RACIAL DIFFERENCES IN HOSPITAL RECORDS, BY HOSPITAL SIZE AND REGION: PAS HOSPITALS, 1968

Hospital Size	East	Midwest	South	West
Small (1-99 beds)	1. Consultations	1. Urinalysis 2. Funduscopic exam. 3. Consultations 4. Antibiotics	1. Urinalysis 2. HGB/HCT exam. 3. Rectal exam. 4. Funduscopic exam.	1. Pelvic exam.
Medium (100-399 beds)	1. Discharges 2. Urinalysis 3. HGB/HCT exam. 4. Rectal exam. 5. Pelvic exam. 6. Parenteral fluids 7. Hosp. infection	1. Death 2. Urinalysis 3. HGB/HCT exam. 4. Pelvic exam. 5. No. elec. determ.	1. Death 2. Urinalysis 3. HGB/HCT exam. 4. Rectal exam. 5. Funduscopic exam. 6. Consultations 7. Antibiotics	1. HGB/HCT exam.
Large (400 + beds)	1. Autopsy 2. Discharges 3. Urinalysis 4. HGB/HCT exam. 5. Rectal exam. 6. Funduscopic exam. 7. Consultations 8. Parenteral fluids	1. Death 2. Discharges 3. Urinalysis 4. HCB/HCT exam. 5. Rectal exam. 6. Pelvic exam. 7. Total consult. 8. Parenteral fluids 9. Complications	1. Discharges 2. Urinalysis 3. HGB/HCT exam. 4. Rectal exam. 5. Pelvic exam. 6. Funduscopic exam. 7. Consultations 8. Parenteral fluids 9. Complications	None

SOURCE: Clayton T. Shaw, "A Detailed Examination of Treatment Procedures of Whites and Blacks in Hospitals," Social Science and Medicine 5 (1971), p. 254. The data were for hospitals participating in the Professional Activity Study and were provided by the Commission on Professional and Hospital Activities in Ann Arbor, Michigan. Shaw examined hospital discharge data on patients in 44 diagnostic groups and sought racial differences in 15 different measures (such as percentage of patients that died, that had a hemoglobin or hematocrit analysis, that had a consultation, that received parenteral fluids but had no electrolyte determination, and that had a hospital infection). Shaw's presentation of the data does not indicate the direction of the statistically significant differences.

important, because of the possibility that minority groups may be underserved or treated differentially, some approaches that focus more heavily on outcome are also potentially useful.

Rutstein et al. have suggested a method that might be applied to examining the outcomes of care as a measure of quality.[154] They postulate that "sentinel events" can often be identified that represent preventable disease, disability, or untimely deaths. Under the approach they describe, the occurrence of these events triggers an investigation in which the responsibility may be determined and corrective action taken. They point to the example of child and maternal health, in which every maternal or perinatal death would lead to an investigation of the prior events to determine what, if anything, went wrong and what steps should be taken to avoid such outcomes. It is clear that not all such deaths are the result of inappropriate or unacceptable care, but enough have been documented and enough changes have been made to significantly lower maternal and perinatal death rates.

By the same logic, documented racial/ethnic differences in the occurrence of "sentinel events" that represent preventable disease, disability, and untimely deaths would be important evidence that unequal, inequitable, and possibly discriminatory care was being given. It is not difficult to identify a number of sentinel events that might be investigated. Decubitus ulcers, infection associated with intrauterine devices, morbidity and mortality associated with various forms of treatable cancers, and the complications of poorly managed intravenous techniques are just a few examples. Most hospitals already monitor such events as post-surgical complications and transfusion reactions, and professional standards review organizations (PSROs) sometimes conduct studies in which racial comparisons could be made in measures of quality of care.

Apparently, no research on racial/ethnic differences has been published based on such an approach. However, some "sentinel events" could be studied using currently available data systems, such as those that exist at the Health Care Financing Administration for Medicare patients and in certain states for Medicaid patients and those at PSROs for both types of patients. If racial/ethnic differences are small, multi-institutional studies will be required. If they are great, differences might be identified within individual institutions. Data from the National Center for Health Statistics Hospital Discharge Survey might also prove amenable to such research.

Three points should be made concerning this approach. First, the study design must account for differences other than race and ethnicity, such as age, sex, income, and severity of illness. Second, differences in the rates of occurrence of sentinel events may be based on racial factors rather than on the medical care that is provided. Even so, such differences may point to differing medical care requirements. Third, as technology advances and practices change, the "sentinel events" (the criteria) may require change, as may the acceptable level of occurrence (the standard).

Hypertension provides an excellent illustration of the last two points. Recent studies clearly show that we have developed a technology to control blood pressure, and, further, that the successful application of this technology results in a significant decrease in morbidity and mortality, even for people with minimally elevated levels, and that these benefits were most pronounced among blacks.[155] It is reasonable to expect that the application of this knowledge will lead to a decrease in strokes and hypertensive cardiovascular disease. It is also known that the incidence and severity of hypertension is greater among middle-aged black males than among others of similar age. This racial difference has more to do with race and sex *per se* than with differences in medical care. However, recognition of this fact should lead to the application of more resources to this unmet need. Thus, monitoring of the impact of this new technology should show a greater impact on morbidity and mortality among blacks than among whites.

Dental Care

Some of the best-documented racial differences in health status are in dental health. Data on treated and untreated dental disease are available through the dental examinations that have been conducted as part of the National Health and Nutritional Survey by the National Center for Health Statistics and are based on sound, representative samples of the U.S. population. As Table 13 shows, consistent racial differences exist in needs for dental treatment (that is, in untreated dental disease). The differences are smallest for the youngest children, but even in the category of age 1-5, black children (5 percent) were more than twice as likely as white children (2 percent) to need dental care to "remove debris and calculus."[156] Among older children and adults, the rates of untreated disease are much higher, and the percentage differences by race are much larger. For example, among blacks aged 12-17, 75 percent had untreated tooth decay, compared to 48 percent of whites. Among blacks aged 65-74, 20 percent needed extractions because of periodontal disease, compared with 7 percent of whites.

Despite evidence showing greater needs for dental treatment among blacks than among whites, national data from the Health Interview Survey show that whites use the services of dentists more than do "other races."[157] As Table 14 shows, this can be partially explained by differences in income, particularly since public funding of dental care is very limited, but racial differences exist even within income categories. Although fewer data are available, there is also evidence of low levels of dental care among the Chicano population.[158]

The explanation of the striking racial discrepancies regarding need and use of service in the dental area is not clear. There are some indications that "discretionary" health services in general are less likely to be used by blacks than by whites; thus, use of dentists in the black population is more confined to the treatment of relatively serious conditions than is true in the white population.[159] However, in at least some parts of the country, the explanation may involve

Table 13. PERCENT OF PERSONS WITH DENTAL TREATMENT NEEDS, BY TYPE OF TREATMENT, AGE AND RACE, 1971-74

Type of Treatment	Total	Age Group: 1 to 5		6 to 11		12 to 17		18 to 64		65 to 74	
		White	Black	White	Black	White	Black	White	Black	White	Black
Number of Persons[1]	191,975	14,220	2,519	19,707	3,458	21,063	3,381	102,997	11,917	11,573	1,138
Percent Needing at Least One Treatment Listed Below	64.1	15.9	19.9	62.2	71.5	64.5	84.7	68.5	90.4	59.5	75.2
Removal of Debris and Calculus	36.7	2.0	5.1	28.8	36.4	38.6	64.0	40.3	67.1	23.9	27.5
Gingivitis Treatment	17.2	--	0.1	1.6	3.8	13.6	24.7	21.3	42.6	13.3	19.0
Periodontal Treatment	10.0	--	0.1	0.1	0.2	1.4	5.8	13.1	26.9	14.1	17.7
Decay, Permanent Teeth	36.9	0.1	0.8	28.8	40.6	48.4	75.5	39.7	65.5	16.6	32.5
Decay, Primary Teeth	6.6	15.4	19.1	39.7	42.4	3.5	1.7	--	--	--	--
Extractions due to Periodontal Disease	2.7	--	--	--	--	--	--	3.0	8.5	6.8	20.1
Fixed Bridges/Partial Removable Dentures	16.0	--	--	0.2	0.1	5.0	9.1	23.3	36.0	8.0	14.2
Other	3.0	0.1	--	0.5	0.1	0.6	0.5	3.8	8.7	3.6	12.4

[1]Population in thousands.

SOURCE: Health and Nutrition Examination Survey (HANES), National Center for Health Statistics (Institute of Medicine, Public Policy Options for Better Dental Health, 1980, p. 17).

Table 14. PERCENT OF PERSONS WITH A DENTAL VISIT WITHIN A YEAR, BY RACE AND INCOME, 1977

Income Level	White	Other Races
Under $5,000	35.4	29.9
$5,000-9,999	38.9	34.3
$10,000 & Over	58.6	41.9

SOURCE: Health Interview Survey, National Center for Health Statistics (Institute of Medicine, Public Policy Options for Better Dental Care, 1980, p. 21).

racial discrimination. The authors of a study of dental care in a rural North Carolina county (where whites reported twice as many dental visits as blacks) attribute part of the large racial difference to the "slow to change established pattern of private health care delivery in Durham County--a certain reluctance on the part of both providers and patients to expand service patterns between like race to those of opposite race when resources are scarce."[160] The extent to which this explanation may account for the national racial patterns in dental care is unknown.

CONCLUSION

From the information described in this chapter, the committee drew the following general conclusions.

First, there is considerable evidence that racial/ethnic factors continue to influence patterns of health care in ways that are not in the interests of the groups that are affected. These patterns are consistent with the belief that minority groups are still exposed to discrimination in this country, although little direct evidence is available.

Second, racial/ethnic patterns in health care deserve much more serious and systematic attention than they have received to date from researchers and governmental statistical agencies. More studies are needed that empirically examine the factors that influence the medical care decisions of minority group members. In recent years, the National Center for Health Statistics and the National Center for Health Services Research have shown more concern with collecting data that will be statistically valid for members of minority groups.[161] Such data are expensive to collect because of sampling problems, yet they are of great importance if equity questions in American health care are to be assessed. The present Health Care Financing Administration (HCFA) data are so inadequate that it is virtually impossible to draw meaningful conclusions about racial/ethnic equity in the Medicaid, Medicare, and Title V programs. HCFA should extend strong efforts to improve the quality of the racial/ethnic information that is collected on beneficiaries of these crucially important federal financing programs. The agreement that was signed between HCFA and OCR in 1980 may be the first step in increasing HCFA's attention to racial and ethnic issues in Medicare and Medicaid.[162]

Third, the question of racial separation in health care and associated questions regarding quality of health care also deserve much more serious attention than they have received to date. At present, many federal policies do not encourage racial/ethnic integration in health care. Since members of some minority groups are disproportionately dependent upon Medicaid, policies that encourage the segregation of Medicaid patients also encourage racial/ethnic segregation. There is little indication that racial separation and the question of separate-but-equal have received serious consideration.

Fourth, specific attention should be given to the factors that may explain the striking racial patterns regarding dental care. The data clearly show that the need for dental care (as defined by untreated disease) is much greater among blacks than among whites, while the use of dental services is much greater among whites than among blacks. Existing data suggest that these trends are due to more than socioeconomic differences.

REFERENCES

1. Hattie Mae Campbell et al. v. R. J. Mincey, Appeal filed with the U.S. Court of Appeals for the Fifth Circuit, No. 76-1325; Geraldine Dallek, "Summary: Health Care for California's Poor: Separate and Unequal," (Santa Monica, CA: National Health Law Program, 1979); Donald Donati, Sylvia Drew Ivie, and Beth Lief, Letter to Harry P. Cain, Bureau of Health Planning and Resources Development, DHEW, October 7, 1977; Carmen Estrada, (Mexican American Legal Defense Fund, San Francisco) Testimony before the Institute of Medicine Committee on Health Care of Minority Groups and Handicapped Persons, Los Angeles, CA, May 9, 1980; Georgia Legal Services et al., "Testimony on Behalf of Legal Services Clients before the Subcommittee on Health and the Environment of the House Committee on Interstate and Foreign Commerce Regarding the Health Planning and Resources Development Amendments of 1978 (H.R. 10460) and Title III of the Hospital Cost Containment Act of 1977 (H.R. 9717)," February 1, 1978; Sylvia Drew Ivie, Ben Thomas Cole, and Beth Lief, Letter to Harry P. Cain, Bureau of Health Planning and Resource Development, DHEW, and to David Tatel, Director, Office for Civil Rights, DHEW, November 7, 1977; Sylvia Drew Ivie and Howard Newman, Joint memorandum from the Director, Office for Civil Rights, and the Administrator, Health Care Financing Administration on "Civil Rights Responsibilities," August 28, 1980; Dorothy T. Lang, Letter to Rep. Charles Rangel, Subcommittee on Health, Committee on Ways

and Means, U.S. House of Representatives, March 24, 1980; Mexican American Legal Defense and Educational Fund v. Madera Community Hospital, Administrative complaint filed with the U.S. Department of Health, Education, and Welfare by Carmen Estrada for the Mexican American Legal Defense and Educational Fund, San Francisco, CA, September 5, 1979; Maria Carmen Ordonez et al. v. Mercy Hospital of Laredo, Administrative complaint filed with the U.S. Department of Health, Education, and Welfare by Lee J. Train for the Texas Rural Legal Aid, Inc., Laredo, TX, April 8, 1980; "Patient Dumping," Investigative series published in the Long Beach Independent Press-Telegram, July 6-16, 1980; Anne Ronan, Letter to Mr. Peter Schey, Director, Alien Rights Center, Legal Aid Foundation of Los Angeles, March 21, 1980; State of California Department of Health, Transcript of Civil Rights Hearing held in Los Angeles, CA, November 14, 1976.

2. Carmen Estrada (Mexican American Legal Defense Fund, San Francisco, CA), Testimony before the Institute of Medicine Committee on Health Care of Minority Groups and Handicapped Persons, Los Angeles, CA, May 9, 1980.
3. Sylvia Drew Ivie, "Ending Discrimination in Health Care: A Dream Deferred," Presentation before the U.S. Civil Rights Commission, April 15, 1980.
4. Sylvia Drew Ivie, Ben Thomas Cole, and Beth Lief, Letter to Harry P. Cain, Bureau of Health Planning and Resource Development, DHEW, and to David Tatel, Director, Office for Civil Rights, DHEW, November 7, 1977.
5. Ivie, pp. 29-30.
6. Bonnie Bullough and Vern L. Bullough, Poverty, Ethnic Identity and Health Care (New York: Appleton, 1972); Paul B. Cornely, "Segregation and Discrimination in Medical Care in the United States," American Journal of Public Health 46 (September 1956) pp. 1074-1081; Herbert M. Morais, The History of the Negro in Medicine (New York: Publishers Co., 1971); Dietrich C. Rietzes, Negroes and Medicine (Cambridge, MA: Harvard University Press, 1958).
7. Kenneth Wing, "Title VI and Health Facilities: Forms Without Substance," Hastings Law Journal 30 (September 1978) p. 145.
8. Bullough and Bullough, p. 162.
9. Wing, pp. 154-161.
10. David E. Hayes-Bautista, "Identifying 'Hispanic' Populations: The Influence of Research Methodology Upon Public Policy," American Journal of Public Health 70 (April 1980) pp. 353-356.
11. Department of Health, Education and Welfare, Health United States: 1979, DHEW Publication No. (PHS) 80-1232 (Washington, D.C.: Government Printing Office, 1980) p. 3.
12. Karen Davis and Cathy Schoen, Health and the War on Poverty: A Ten-Year Appraisal (Washington, D.C.: The Brookings Institution, 1978) p. 1.
13. Lu Ann Aday, Ronald Andersen, and Gretchen V. Fleming, Health Care in the U.S.: Equitable for Whom? (Beverly Hills, CA: Sage, 1980) p. 18.

14. U.S. Department of Health, Education, and Welfare, Health United States: 1979, p. 3.
15. Davis and Schoen, p. 1.
16. Aday, Andersen, and Fleming, p. 18.
17. Health Care Financing Administration, "Medicaid State Tables, 1977" (Unpublished data, 1980).
18. Health United States: 1979, p. 15.
19. Ibid., p. 17.
20. Melvin H. Rudov and Nancy Santangelo, Health Status of Minorities and Low-Income Groups, DHEW Publication No. (HRA) 79-627 (Washington, D.C.: Government Printing Office, 1979) p. 36.
21. Lester Breslow and Bonnie Klein, "Health and Race in California," Journal of the American Public Health Association 61 (April 1971) p. 769.
22. Health Resources Administration, Health of the Disadvantaged: Chartbook, DHEW Publication No. (HRA) 77-628 (Washington, D.C.: DHEW, 1977); K. S. Markides, H. W. Martin, and E. Gomez, "Older Mexican Americans: A Study in an Urban Barrio," Chapter 6: Health Status and Health Care Utilization, Unpublished manuscript; Chicano Health Institute of Students, Professors, and Alumni, The California Raza Health Plan: An Action Guide for the Promotion of Raza Health in California (Berkeley, CA, CHISPA: 1979).
23. Health United States: 1979, p. 21.
24. Ibid.
25. Jerry L. Weaver, National Health Policy and the Underserved: Ethnic Minorities, Women, and the Elderly (St. Louis, MO: Mosby, 1976) p. 60; Ian Canino, Brian Earley, and Lloyd Rogler, The Puerto Rican Child in New York City: Stress and Mental Health. (Bronx, NY: Fordham University Hispanic Research Center, 1980).
26. Mary Grace Kovar, "Mortality of Black Infants in the United States," Phylon 38 (December 1977) p. 389.
27. Health United States: 1979, pp. 140-141.
28. Ibid., p. 25.
29. Rudov and Santangelo, pp. 91-92.
30. Lillian M. Axtell, Ardyce J. Asire, and Max H. Myers (eds.), Cancer Patient Survival, Report No. 5 from the Cancer Surveillance, Epidemiology and End Results (SEER) Program, DHEW Publication No. (NIH) 77-992 (Washington, D.C.: Government Printing Office, 1977) p. 4.
31. Ibid., p. 5.
32. Ibid., p. 9.
33. Ibid.
34. Jack E. White et al., "Cancer Among Blacks in the United States--Recognizing the Problem," To be published in the Proceedings of the International Conference on Cancer among Black Populations, held at Roswell Park Memorial Institute, Buffalo, NY, May 5 and 6, 1980, p. 10.
35. Earl S. Pollock and John W. Horm, "Trends in Cancer Incidence and Mortality in the United States, 1969-76," Journal of the National Cancer Institute 64 (May 1980) p. 1101.

36. Donald Fredrickson, Testimony before the House of Representatives Subcommittee on Health and the Environment, Committee on Interstate and Foreign Commerce, June 18, 1979.
37. Health United States: 1979, p. 25; National Diabetes Data Group "Selected Statistics on Health and Medical Care of Diabetics, 1980," forthcoming.
38. National Diabetes Data Group; Rudov and Santangelo, pp. 114 and 118; Department of Health, Education, and Welfare, "VD Fact Sheet - 1971"; Center for Disease Control, 1978 Tuberculosis Statistics: States and Cities, DHEW Publication No. (CDC) 80-8249 (Washington, D.C.: DHEW, 1979).
39. Pollock and Horm, pp. 1093-1094.
40. Rudov and Santangelo, p. 110; National Center for Health Statistics, Prevalence of Selected Chronic Respiratory Conditions, United States-1970, Vital and Health Statistics, Series 10, No. 84, (Washington, D.C.: Government Printing Office, 1973); National Center for Health Statistics, Prevalence of Chronic Skin and Musculoskeletal Conditions, United States-1969, Vital and Health Statistics, Series 10, No. 92, (Washington, D.C.: DHEW, 1974).
41. National Center for Health Statistics, Prevalence of Selected Chronic Respiratory Conditions, United States-1970, Vital and Health Statistics, Series 10, No. 84. (Washington, D.C.: Government Printing Office, 1973) p. 15; National Center for Health Statistics, Prevalence of Chronic Skin and Musculoskeletal Conditions, United States-1969, Vital and Health Statistics, Series 10, No. 92, (Washington, D.C.: DHEW, 1974); National Center for Health Statistics, Prevalence of Selected Chronic Digestive Conditions: United States, 1975, Vital and Health Statistics, Series 10, No. 123. (Washington, D.C.: DHEW, 1979).
42. Health United States: 1979, p. 127.
43. Health Resources Administration, Health of the Disadvantaged: Chartbook, p. 33; California Raza Health Plan, pp. 35 and 41.
44. Jose Oscar Alers, Puerto Ricans and Health: Findings from New York City (Bronx, NY: Fordham University Hispanic Research Center, 1978).
45. Robert E. Roberts and Eun Sul Lee, "The Health of Mexican Americans: Evidence from the Human Population Laboratory Studies," American Journal of Public Health 70 (April 1980) pp. 375-384.
46. David Mechanic, Medical Sociology, Second Edition (New York: Free Press, 1978) pp. 273-287.
47. Sandra Green, Eva Salber, and Jacob J. Feldman, "Distribution of Illness and Its Implications in a Rural Community," Medical Care 14 (December 1978) p. 872.
48. Health United States: 1979, pp. 37-38.
49. Ibid., pp. 37-39.
50. Marjorie Cantor and Mary Mayer, "Health and the Inner City Elderly," The Gerontologist 16 (1976) p. 19; Deborah Newquist et al., Prescription for Neglect: Experience of Older Blacks and

Mexican-Americans with the American Health Care System, Final Report on Administration on Aging Grant No. 90-A-1297 (Los Angeles, CA: Andrus Gerontology Center, 1979); J. J. Dowd and V. L. Benston, "Aging in Minority Populations: An Examination of the Double Jeopardy Hypothesis," Journal of Gerontology 33 (1978) pp. 417-436; Markides et al., pp. 8-14.
51. Ethel Shanas, National Survey of the Aged, Final Report of Social Security Administration Contract No. 10P-57823, (no date); Newquist et al.; Cantor and Mayer, p. 19.
52. Dorothy Rice and Kathleen M. Danchik, "Changing Needs of Children: Disease, Disability and Access to Care," Presented at the Annual Meeting of the Institute of Medicine, October 25, 1979.
53. Rice and Danchik, Table 7; Health United States: 1979, p. 37.
54. Health United States: 1979, p. 37.
55. Ibid., p. 9.
56. Rudov and Santangelo, p. 87.
57. Select Panel for the Promotion of Child Health, Better Health for Our Children: A National Strategy, 4 vols., (Washington, D.C.: Government Printing Office, 1980).
58. Health United States: 1979, p. 187.
59. Eva S. Salber et al., "Access to Health Care in a Southern Rural Community," Medical Care 14 (December 1976) pp. 971-986.
60. Aday, Andersen, and Fleming, p. 106.
61. Diana Dutton, "Children's Health Care: The Myth of Equal Access," Background paper prepared for the Select Panel for the Promotion of Child Health, July 1980.
62. Ibid., Tables 7 and 8.
63. Ibid.
64. National Center for Health Statistics, Office Visits by Women. The National Ambulatory Medical Care Survey, United States, 1977, Vital and Health Statistics, Series 13, No. 45. (Washington, D.C.: DHEW, 1980) p. 10.
65. Ibid.
66. National Center for Health Statistics, unpublished tables from the 1978 Health Interview Survey.
67. Alers, pp. 31-55; Weaver, p. 63.
68. Research evidence leaves some doubt about the exact role that prenatal care may play in influencing infant mortality figures. Although groups that receive little or no prenatal care have higher infant mortality rates, questions of causation remain. Low birth weight is generally acknowledged to be the major risk factor for infant mortality, and the higher incidence of low birth weight infants among blacks is amply documented and is true regardless of age, marital status, and receipt of prenatal care (NCHS, Series 21, Number 37). Furthermore, evidence that prenatal care influences birth weight is ambiguous, at best. The incidence of low birth weight hardly varied no matter when, in the course of pregnancy, prenatal care was undertaken (NCHS, Series 21, No. 37, 1980: 16). That is, there is little difference in rates of low birth weight between women who

initiated prenatal care in the first or second month of pregnancy and women who initiated prenatal care in the seventh to ninth months of pregnancy. This is true regardless of factors such as race, age, and marital status. However, the incidence of low birth weight infants is greatly elevated among women who receive no prenatal care (a category that includes disproportionate numbers of blacks), although causation is not clear. In many cases it appears that both the low birth weight and the lack of prenatal care are a result of the prematurity of the birth (NCHS, Series 31, No. 33: 21).

69. National Center for Health Statistics, Prenatal Care; United States, 1969-1975, Vital and Health Statistics, Series 31, No. 33, (Washington, D.C.: DHEW, 1978).
70. Ibid., pp. 14-17.
71. Ibid., p. 14.
72. Ibid., p. 19.
73. Mary Grace Kovar, "Mortality of Black Infants in the United States," Phylon 38 (December 1977) pp. 370-397.
74. Aday, Andersen, and Fleming, p. 118.
75. Antonio S. Medina, "Hispanic Reproductive Health in California, 1976-77," Paper presented at annual meeting of the American Public Health Association, 1979.
76. The "use-disability" ratio is:

$$\frac{P}{D} \times 100,$$

where P is the mean number of physician visits for those with one or more disability days, and D is the mean number of disability days for those with one or more disability days.

The "symptoms-response" ratio reflects a degree of medical judgment about the need for medical care in the presence of various symptoms. The actual ratio is:

$$\frac{A-E}{E} \times 100,$$

where A is the actual number of persons who contact a doctor at least once for given symptoms, and E is the estimate of a panel of physicians of the number of persons who should contact a doctor for those symptoms (Aday, Andersen, and Fleming, 1980, pp. 186, 192-193).

77. Problems with the symptoms-response ratio include its disregard of preventive care, its dependence on respondent recognition and reports of symptoms, and its disregard of the severity of and interaction among symptoms. See Dutton, p. 22; Ronald Andersen, "Health Status Indices and Access to Medical Care," American Journal of Public Health 68 (May 1978) p. 461; Martin K. Chen, "Comment on 'Health Status Indices and Access to Medical Care,' " American Journal of Public Health 68 (October 1978)

p. 1027. Some believe that these problems lead to overestimates of the poor's use of medical care in relation to symptoms. Some of the same problems (for example, the disregard of prevention) and analagous problems (there may be class or ethnic differences in what is defined as disability) also apply to the use-disability ratio. The problems with these measures are acknowledged and discussed in reports of the most recent research (Aday, Andersen, and Fleming, 1980, pp. 192-196).

78. Andersen, p. 461; Aday, Andersen, and Fleming, p. 195.
79. Aday, Andersen, and Fleming, p. 197.
80. Andersen; Dutton, p. 24; Aday, Andersen and Fleming, p. 983.
81. National Center for Health Statistics, Use of Selected Medical Procedures Associated with Preventive Care: United States--1973, Vital and Health Statistics, Series 10, No. 110. (Washington, D.C.: DHEW, 1977) p. 27.
82. Aday, Andersen, and Fleming, p. 116.
83. Roberts and Lee.
84. Aday, Andersen, and Fleming, p. 76.
85. Roberts and Lee.
86. Salber et al., p. 190.
87. Stephen Thacker et al., "Primary Health Care in an Academic Medical Center," American Journal of Public Health 68 (September 1978) p. 69.
88. Mildred A. Morehead, "Evaluating Quality of Medical Care in the Neighborhood Health Center Program of the Office of Economic Opportunity," Medical Care 8 (March-April 1970) p. 130.
89. National Center for Health Statistics, "Advance Data, Health Interview Survey 1974," DHEW Publication No. (PHS) 78-1250, 1978.
90. Aday, Andersen, and Fleming, p. 59.
91. Ibid.
92. Health United States: 1979, p. 7.
93. Aday, Andersen, and Fleming, p. 89.
94. Davis and Schoen; Aday, Andersen, and Fleming; Rudov and Santangelo; E. A. Skinner et al., "Use of Ambulatory Health Services by the Near Poor," American Journal of Public Health 68 (1978) pp. 1195-1201.
95. S. W. Shannon and G. E. A. Dever, Health Care Delivery: Spatial Perspectives (New York: McGraw Hill, 1974).
96. Alers.
97. David Elesh and Paul T. Schollaert, "Race and Urban Medicine: Factors Affecting the Distribution of Physicians in Chicago," Journal of Health and Social Behavior 13 (September 1972) pp. 236-250; Robert S. Kaplan and Samuel Leinhardt, "Determinants of Physician Office Location," Medical Care 11 (September 1973) pp. 406-415.
98. Elesh and Schollaert; Guzick and Jahiel, "Distribution of Private Practice Offices of Physicians with Specified Characteristics Among Urban Neighborhoods," Medical Care 14 (June 1976) pp. 419-488.
99. Guzick and Jahiel.

100. Alfred E. Miller, "The Changing Structure of the Medical Profession in Urban and Suburban Settings," Social Science and Medicine 11 (1977) pp. 233-243.
101. Pierre Devise, Misused and Misplaced Hospitals and Doctors: A Locational Analysis of the Urban Health Care Crisis (Washington, D.C.: Association of American Geographers, 1973).
102. Louise M. Okada and Gerald Sparer, "Access to Usual Source of Care by Race and Income in Ten Urban Areas," Journal of Community Health 1 (Spring 1976) pp. 163-174.
103. Ed Bradley, "Blacks in America: With All Deliberate Speed?" CBS Television, (July 24, 1979); Karen Davis and Ray Marshall, "Section 1502(l). Primary Health Care Services for Medically Underserved Populations," in Papers on the National Health Guidelines: The Priorities of Section 1502 (Washington, D.C.: DHEW, 1977) pp. 14-23; Aaron Shirley, Presentation before the U.S. Civil Rights Commission on the federal role in rural health care delivery, April 15, 1980, p. 3.
104. Theodore D. Wood, Office of Civilian Health and Medical Programs of the Uniformed Services, Department of Defense, Letter of finding to William Baxter, Administrator, Newnan Hospital, Newnan, Georgia, November 19, 1979.
105. Janet B. Mitchell and Jerry Cromwell, Large Medicaid Practices: Are They Medicaid Mills? Health Care Financing Grants and Contracts Report Series (Washington, D.C.: DHEW, 1980) p. 41.
106. Ibid., pp. 33 and 38.
107. Ibid., p. 43.
108. The Physician Capacity Utilization Surveys: Health Manpower References, DHEW Publication No. (HRA) 79-30, (Washington, D.C.: DHEW, 1979).
109. Davis and Marshall, p. 14.
110. Frank E. Moss, "Through the Medicaid Mills," The Journal of Legal Medicine 5 (May 1977) pp. 6-11, reprinted in Alan D. Spiegel (ed.), The Medicaid Experience (Germantown, MD: Aspen, 1979) pp. 387-392.
111. Institute of Medicine, Assessing Quality in Health Care: An Evaluation (Washington, D.C.: National Academy of Sciences, 1976).
112. Robert H. Brook and Kathleen N. Williams, "Quality of Health Care for the Disadvantaged," Journal of Community Medicine 1 (Winter 1975) pp. 132-156.
113. Rodney M. Coe and H. P. Brehm, "Preventive Health Services and Physician Error," Social Science and Medicine 7 (1973) pp. 303-305.
114. B. A. Lockett and K. N. Williams, Foreign Medical Graduates and Physician Manpower in the United States, DHEW Publication No. (HRA) 74-30 (Washington, D.C.: Government Printing Office, 1974).
115. Mitchell and Cromwell, p. 42.
116. Frank Sloan, Janet Mitchell, and Jerry Cromwell, "Physician Participation in State Medicaid Programs," The Journal of Human Resources 13 (Supplement, 1978) pp. 211-245; Mitchell and Cromwell; F. Kavaler, "Medicaid in New York: Utopianism and Bare

Knuckles in Public Health. IV. People, Providers and Payment Telling How It Is," American Journal of Public Health 59 (May 1969) pp. 820-825; Michael W. Jones and Bette Hamburger, "A Survey of Physician Participation in and Dissatisfaction with the Medi-Cal Program," The Western Journal of Medicine 124 (January 1976) pp. 75-83; reprinted in Alan D. Spiegel (ed.), The Medicaid Experience, (Germantown, MD: Aspen, 1979) pp. 277-289.

117. Sloan, Mitchell, and Cromwell, James Studnicki, Robert M. Saywell, Walter Wiechetek, "Foreign Medical Graduates and Maryland Medicaid," New England Journal of Medicine 294 (1976) pp. 1153-1157, reprinted in Alan D. Spiegel (ed.), The Medicaid Experience (Germantown, MD: Aspen, 1979).
118. Kavaler; Alers.
119. Alers.
120. Lawrence S. Bloom et al., "Medicaid in Cook County: Present Status and Future Prospects," Inquiry 5 (June 1968) pp. 13-23.
121. Mitchell and Cromwell, p. 113.
122. Ibid.
123. Aday, Andersen, and Fleming, pp. 157, 160.
124. Ibid.
125. Barbara S. Hulka et al., "Correlates of Satisfaction and Dissatisfaction with Medical Care: A Community Perspective," Medical Care 8 (August 1975) pp. 648-658.
126. Aday, Andersen, and Fleming, pp. 144-148.
127. Ibid., p. 122; Health United States: 1979, pp. 40-42.
128. Health United States: 1979, p. 40; Rudov and Santangelo, p. 239; National Center for Health Statistics, Utilization of Short-Stay Hospitals: Annual Summary for the United States, 1978, Vital and Health Statistics, Series 13, No 46. (Washington, D.C.: DHEW, 1980) p. 46.
129. Rudov and Santangelo, p. 244.
130. National Center for Health Statistics, Utilization of Short-Stay Hospitals: Annual Summary for the United States, 1978, Vital and Health Statistics, Series 13, No. 46. (Washington, D.C.: DHEW, 1980) p. 46.
131. Center for Disease Control, Surgical Sterilization Surveillance: Tubal Sterilization 1970-1975, DHEW Publication No. (CDC) 79-8378 (Atlanta, GA: CDC, 1979) p. 13.
132. Ibid.
133. National Center for Health Statistics, National Survey of Family Growth (Unpublished data).
134. Center for Disease Control, Surgical Sterilization Surveillance: Tubal Sterilization 1970-1975, p. 13.
135. Subcommittee on Health of the Committee on Labor and Public Welfare, United States Senate, Hearings on Quality of Health Care--Human Experimentation, 1973, Part 4. (Washington, D.C.: Government Printing Office, 1973).
136. Bradford H. Gray, Human Subjects in Medical Experimentation (New York: Wiley-Interscience, 1975).

137. Peter M. Layde et al. "Demographic Trends of Tubal Sterilization in the United States, 1970-1975" (Unpublished) p. 5.
138. Devise.
139. Ibid., p. 25
140. Pierre Devise, "Persistence of Chicago's Dual Hospital System," in Pierre Devise (ed.) Slum Medicine: Chicago's Apartheid Health System (Chicago: Community and Family Study Center, University of Chicago, 1969) p. 19.
141. Ibid., p.24.
142. Richard L. Morrill, Robert S. Earickson, and Philip Rees, "Factors Influencing Distance Traveled to Hospitals," Economic Geography 46 (April 1970) pp. 161-170.
143. R. L. Bashur, G. W. Shannon, and C. M. Metzner,"Some Ecological Differentials in the Use of Medical Services, "Health Services Research 6 (Spring 1971).
144. Ibid., p. 69.
145. General Counsel of DHEW et al., Brief submitted in the matters of: Mercy Hospital, Southern Baptist Hospital, Hotel Dieu Hospital et al., DHEW Docket Numbers 78-VI-7, 78-VI-8, and 78-VI-9 (1978).
146. Numerous indices or summary measures of spatial or organizational segregation have been proposed and evaluated, especially within the sociological literature. These measures have often been applied as indices of the extent to which a residential or school system population is racially segregated. Most widely used has been the "index of dissimilarity," which provides a measure of the extent to which a "system" as a whole is segregated (or integrated) based upon the extent to which the racial composition of each unit of measurement (school, census tract, hospital, etc.) deviates from a theoretical norm at which the percent black and percent white of each unit would be the same as the overall percentage of each group within the system as a whole. For interpretative purposes, this index "D" can also be considered as the percentage of the minority (or non-minority) population that would have to be redistributed were each unit were to have the identical racial makeup. See Otis and Beverly Duncan, "A Methodological Analysis of Segregation Indices," American Sociological Review 20 (April 1955) pp. 210-217.
147. Raymond S. Duff and August B. Hollingshead, Sickness and Society (New York: Harper and Row, 1968).
148. Lawrence D. Egbert and Ilene L. Rothman. "Relation Between the Race and Economic Status of Patients and Who Performs Their Surgery," New England Journal of Medicine 297 (July 14, 1977) pp. 89-91.
149. Joseph A. Flaherty and Robert Meagher, "Measuring Racial Bias in Inpatient Treatment," American Journal of Psychiatry 137 (June 1980) pp. 679-682.
150. Anna M. Jackson, Hershel Berkowitz, and Gordon K. Farley, "Race as a Variable Affecting the Treatment Involvement of Children," Journal of the American Academy of Child Psychiatry 13 (1974) pp. 20-31.

151. Stanley Sue, "Community Mental Health Services to Minority Groups," American Psychologist (August 1977) pp. 616-624.
152. Ibid., pp. 620-621.
153. Clayton T. Shaw, "A Detailed Examination of Treatment Procedures of Whites and Blacks in Hospitals," Social Science and Medicine 5 (1971) pp. 251-256.
154. David D. Rutstein et al., "Measuring the Quality of Medical Care: A Clinical Method," New England Journal of Medicine 294 (March 11, 1976) pp. 582-588.
155. Hypertension Detection and Follow-up Program Cooperative Group, "Five-Year Findings of the Hypertension Detection and Follow-up Program. I. Reduction in Mortality of Persons With High Blood Pressure, Including Mild Hypertension. II. Mortality by Race-Sex and Age," Journal of the American Medical Association 242 (December 1979) pp. 2562-2577.
156. Institute of Medicine, Public Policy Options for Better Dental Health, (Washington, D.C.: National Academy Press, 1980).
157. Ibid.
158. Roberts and Lee, p. 266.
159. Joanna Kravits and John Schneider, "The Relationship of Attitudes to Discretionary Physician and Dentist Use by Race and Income" in Ronald Anderson, Joanna Kravits, and Odin Anderson (eds.), Equity in Health Services: Empirical Analyses in Social Policy (Cambridge, MA: Ballinger, 1975) pp. 169-187.
160. Eva J. Salber et al., "Utilization of Services for Preventable Disease: A Case Study of Dental Care in a Southern Rural Area of the United States," International Journal of Epidemiology 7 (1978) pp. 163-173; Eva J. Salber et al., "Access to Health Care in a Southern Rural Community," Medical Care 14 (December 1976) p. 983.
161. Eva J. Salber and Angell Beza, "The Health Interview Survey and Minority Health," Medical Care 18 (March 1980) pp. 319-326; Dorothy P. Rice, Thomas F. Drury, and Robert H. Mugge, "Household Health Interviews and Minority Health," Medical Care 18 (March 1980) pp. 327-335.
162. Ivie and Newman.

3

RACIAL DIFFERENCES IN USE OF NURSING HOMES

Racial and ethnic variations in the use of nursing homes are a distinct feature of American health care. Elderly blacks* use nursing homes at lower rates than do whites. Various explanations have been offered, including differences in family networks and values, differences in geographic proximity to nursing homes, racial differences in survival and in numbers of elderly people, and racial discrimination. Although the pattern of less black use of nursing homes has been recognized for many years, the committee was unable to locate sufficient data for a definitive sorting out of the competing explanations. Notwithstanding the dearth of information for a direct assessment of discrimination in nursing home admissions, indirect evidence raises the possibility that discrimination may be widespread. However, little attention has been given to documenting it or to bringing civil rights enforcement activities to bear on it.

Evidence pertaining to the racial difference in the use of nursing homes is reviewed in this chapter. Evidence regarding discrimination comes largely from data showing the inadequacy of competing explanations. To summarize this evidence, the low use of nursing homes by blacks is apparent in <u>rates</u> of nursing home use, not only in numbers (which may be affected by differential mortality rates). All indications are that the health problems and disabilities that create the need for nursing home care are at least as common among blacks as whites, and, although some differences in family living arrangements

---

*The emphasis of this chapter is on the use of nursing homes by the black elderly. This is the ethnic minority about which the most concern has been expressed regarding possible discrimination in nursing homes, and it is the minority about which the most adequate data exist. Although there is a growing body of literature about the elderly in other minority groups, it is not adequate for a description of patterns of nursing home use and possible causes for patterns that are distinct to particular ethnic groups. The problems of explanation that are reviewed in this chapter are less difficult than the problems that would be faced in attempting a similar analysis of the use of nursing homes by any other ethnic minority group.

can be documented, there is no indication that partially disabled, elderly whites are less successful than blacks in securing needed assistance at home. Blacks probably suffer disproportionately from disincentives perceived by nursing homes in accepting Medicaid patients. In addition, there are indications from some states of a large racial difference in meeting the needs for nursing home care of elderly poor persons within the Medicaid population.

Because the federal government, particularly through the Medicaid program, is the major source of money for nursing home care, and this federal involvement triggers the applicability of the Civil Rights Act's prohibition of discrimination, the lack of direct evidence about discrimination in nursing homes is rather remarkable. Similarly, although there is widespread agreement among knowledgeable persons that nursing homes have strong tendencies toward racial segregation, little direct documentation is available, despite all of the claims forms that are submitted for Medicaid and Medicare reimbursement. It is evident that the possibility, even the likelihood, of widespread patterns of discrimination and segregation in nursing homes has not been regarded by government as an important problem.

INTRODUCTION

There are about 18,900 nursing homes* in the United States in which more than 1,300,000 persons, mostly elderly, reside and receive care.[2] Most (77 percent) nursing homes are privately owned, proprietary institutions,[3] and some have religious affiliations. Data are not available on the countless boarding homes that provide some aspect of nursing home care, because few of these homes are licensed. Most come to official attention only when a fire or other disaster occurs.

Although it has been known for years that minority groups make less use of nursing homes than do whites, some doubt may be raised about whether this pattern merits concern, because nursing home care is not an unmixed blessing. As Vladeck noted in his recent examination of nursing homes for the Twentieth Century Fund:

> [Nursing homes] have been described as "Houses of Death," "concentration camps," "warehouses for the dying." It is a documented fact that nursing home residents tend to deteriorate, physically and psychologically, after being

---

*The National Nursing Home Survey includes several categories of nursing homes. The survey is not confined to facilities that are certified for Medicare and Medicaid reimbursment purposes as "skilled nursing facilities" or "intermediate care facilities." Not all homes in the survey actually provided "nursing services;" all, however, provided residents with assistance in activities of daily living.[1]

> placed in what are presumably therapeutic institutions. The overuse of potent medications in nursing homes is a scandal in itself. Thousands of facilities in every state of the nation fail to meet minimal government standards of sanitation, staffing, or patient care. The best governmental estimate is that roughly half the nation's nursing homes are "substandard."[4]

Yet nursing homes meet important individual and societal needs for which adequate alternatives (stipends for family care, day care facilities, respite care, foster care, and so forth) do not widely exist. People reside in nursing homes because they are dependent upon others for some aspects of their care. According to the 1977 National Nursing Home Survey, more than 86 percent of nursing home residents require assistance in bathing, 69 percent require assistance in dressing, 52 percent require assistance in using the toilet room, 66 percent can walk only with assistance or are chairfast or bedfast, 45 percent have difficulty with bowel or bladder control, and 33 percent require assistance with eating.[5] Fewer than 10 percent are dependent in none of the above activities, and almost one-fourth are dependent in all of them. For almost 80 percent of the patients, the primary reason given for residence in nursing homes is care needs stemming from poor physical health; other reasons included mental illness, mental retardation, behavioral problems, and social and economic reasons. For many persons a combination of factors is undoubtedly involved. The median age of patients is 81. Chronic conditions and impairments are common and varied, and include arteriosclerosis (48 percent of residents), hypertension (21 percent), stroke (16 percent), heart trouble (34 percent), chronic brain syndrome (25 percent), and senility (32 percent). A gross measure of the demand for nursing home care is provided by the remarkable growth of the nursing home "industry"--bed capacity tripled between 1954 and 1973 and has continued to grow.[6]

The fact that nursing homes are populated by people who need care does not demonstrate that such care is best provided in nursing homes. It is estimated that between 10 and 40 percent of the elderly placed in nursing homes could be better served, and at a lower cost to the community, were the necessary services available.[7] But adequate domiciliary services are not available. In the face of concerns about cost and quality of nursing home care and the growth of the elderly population, interest in alternatives is growing. At present, however, public policy (as expressed by Medicare and Medicaid) continues to favor inpatient nursing home care.

The fact remains that aging is often accompanied by the development of chronic physical and mental problems that produce a need for assistance. Nursing homes are an important source of such assistance, particularly when the needs for care exceed the capacity of dedicated family members and friends. There is little doubt that the need is genuine and not due to such factors as the shirking of family responsibilities, as seems to be widely believed. As Elaine Brody wrote, "Overall, the responsible behavior of families towards older people has been so thoroughly documented that it is no longer at issue in gerontological research."[8] Much of the use of nursing homes in the past two decades can be accounted for by the growth of the over-75 population (and its substantial number of unmarried women without children) and by the deinstitutionalization movement in mental hospitals that once provided a home for many of the confused elderly.[9]

Thus, because nursing homes have a near monopoly on continuing care of the elderly, and are needed to meet the needs of a population that requires both medical care and assistance in activities of daily living, there is reason for concern about possible inequities in access. A second reason for concern arises from the flow of tax dollars to nursing homes and the consequences of this flow for different members of the population. Public policy decisions are responsible for many of the characteristics of the nursing home industry, both because public money is the dominant source of nursing home dollars and because of the regulatory web that accompanies those public funds.[10] Three-fourths of nursing homes (containing almost 90 percent of nursing home beds) are certified to receive federal monies through the Medicare or Medicaid programs, and the federal dollar is the most important source of payment for nursing home care. Figures for 1976-78 show that the federal government provided 53 percent of the nursing home dollars, mostly through the Medicaid program.[11]

States also are a major source of funds for nursing home care through Medicaid matching funds. Because Medicaid programs are run by the states (with a substantial federal subsidy), state governments can be regarded as large purchasers of nursing home services. In the view of some observers, budgetary pressures at the state level bring the state's self-interest into conflict with the interests of persons needing nursing home care. This conflict is manifested in vigorous restraint of reimbursement rates (with a predictable impact on the availability of beds) and in less than vigorous attention to standards of quality.[12]

USE OF NURSING HOMES BY BLACKS

Questions have long been asked about minority group access to nursing homes. For example, Senator Moss opened a set of hearings on long-term care in 1972 with the question, "Why are there no members of minority groups in nursing homes? It is a fact that comparatively few blacks, Asians, Indians, or Mexican-Americans are in nursing homes."[13] His Subcommittee on Long-Term Care heard testimony about a variety of barriers to nursing home admission for racial or ethnic minorities. There was testimony about the problem of distance from nursing homes for Indians on Arizona reservations, language and cultural barriers for Asian Americans and Mexican Americans, and racism and economic and cultural barriers for blacks. The concerns expressed about the unmet needs of elderly individuals from different racial and ethnic minority groups was paralleled by frustration about the lack of data to document and explain, in a systematic way, ethnic patterns of disparity and unmet needs.

However, a general picture of nursing home use by blacks has been available for some time. National studies have consistently shown low rates of use, although there is evidence of a slow increase.* The underrepresentation of minorities is most clearly seen when different age groups are compared. Table 15 presents data for all age groups over 65 and shows lower rates of nursing home use by non-whites than whites since 1963. Although the non-white rate has increased more rapidly than the white rate since that time, the most recent data still show a very substantial racial difference. Fifty per 1,000 white persons aged 65 and over were residents of nursing homes in 1977, compared with 30 per 1,000 for the rest of the population. Persons 85 years of age and over who are white are twice as likely as others of this age to be receiving nursing home care and the federal and state tax dollars that support it.

Table 15 also shows that the lower black use of nursing homes is not simply due to differential mortality. Although it is true that the number of elderly blacks is smaller than it would be if white and black life expectancy at birth had been equivalent over the past 65 years, this fact does not affect the rates shown in Table 15, because they are stated in terms of the population aged 65 and older. Furthermore, at age 65 there is no longer much difference in life expectancy between whites and others, and in older age categories the mortality rate for whites exceeds that for blacks.[18]

Table 15 also shows that the racial pattern of nursing home use differs among different age groups. In 1977, among persons aged 65-74, the white rate of nursing home use was actually slightly lower than the non-white rate (14.2 versus 16.8 per 1,000). (Whether this pattern will continue as this cohort ages remains to be seen.) However, among those 75-84, the non-white rate was only 55 percent of the white rate, and among those above age 85, the non-white rate was only 45 percent of the white rate. In the latter category, one-fourth of the white population were residents of nursing or personal care homes as compared to only one-tenth of the rest of the population.

---

*The National Center for Health Statistics (NCHS) 1969 survey of residents of "nursing and personal care" homes showed that 4.5 of the residents were from groups other than "whites."[14] The 1973-74 National Nursing Home Survey showed blacks as 4.6 percent of the nursing home population, while "Spanish-American" patients made up 1.1 percent.[15] Comparable figures from the 1977 Nursing Home Survey were 6.2 percent blacks and 1.1 percent "Hispanics."[16] Among persons aged 65 and over, members of racial/ethnic groups other than "white" made up 9 percent of the U.S. population, but only 5.2 percent of the nursing home population in 1973-74.[17] The 1977 survey showed persons from groups other than "whites" to constitute 6.8 percent of nursing home residents aged 65 and over.

Table 15. NURSING HOME AND PERSONAL CARE HOME RESIDENTS 65 YEARS AND OVER, ACCORDING TO AGE AND COLOR

Year and Age	Number of Residents	Number per 1,000 Population	
		White[1]	All Other
1963			
65 years and over	445,600	26.6	10.3
65-74 years	89,600	8.1	5.9
75-84 years	207,200	41.7	13.8
85 years and over	148,700	157.7	41.8
1969			
65 years and over	722,200	38.8	17.6
65-74 years	138,500	11.7	9.6
75-84 years	321,800	54.1	22.9
85 years and over	261,900	221.9	52.4
1973-74[2]			
65 years and over	961,500	48.1	21.9
65-74 years	163,100	12.5	10.6
75-84 years	384,900	61.9	30.1
85 years and over	413,600	269.0	91.4
1977[3]			
65 years and over	1,126,000	49.7	30.4
65-74 years	211,400	14.2	16.8
75-84 years	464,700	70.6	38.6
85 years and over	449,900	229.0	102.0

[1]Includes Hispanics.
[2]Excludes residents in personal care homes.
[3]Includes residents in domiciliary care homes.

SOURCE: Department of Health and Human Services, Health: United States, 1980 (Washington, D.C.: Government Printing Office, 1981) p. 496. Data are based on national surveys of nursing homes conducted by the National Center for Health Statistics in the years shown.

Levels of Disability

If the use of nursing homes was simply a function of degree of disability, there would be more blacks than whites in nursing homes; studies consistently show more disability among elderly blacks than among elderly whites. Table 16, for example, presents responses from household interviews conducted by the National Center for Health Statistics in a national sample of the non-institutionalized population and shows that among those above age 65, blacks were more likely than whites to report limitations in activity and mobility and days of restricted activity and bed disability.[19] Blacks aged 65 and older reported an average of 25 days of bed disability in 1977 compared with an average of 12 days of bed disability for whites in the same age category. Half of the blacks above age 65 reported that they were limited in a major activity, compared with 36 percent of the whites. Twenty-four percent of the blacks reported limitation of mobility, compared with 17 percent of whites.

Similar findings emerged from the 1975 National Survey of the Black Aged sponsored by the Social Security Administration and the Administration on Aging. Shanas summarized the findings on health status:

> 1. Although there is little difference between blacks and whites in their proportions of household and bedfast elderly, black aged, particularly black women, report more restricted physical mobility than do whites. Black women are far more likely than white women to report that they can go outdoors only with difficulty.
>
> 2. Capacity for self-care is less among blacks than among whites. Again, the greatest amount of incapacity is reported by black women.
>
> 3. Blacks are twice as likely as whites to report difficulties with common physical tasks.
>
> 4. Blacks are twice as likely as whites to report that they were giddy at least once during the week before they were interviewed.
>
> 5. Blacks are twice as likely as whites to report that they had spent time ill in bed the year before they were interviewed, and they are more likely than whites to report that they saw a doctor during the month before their interviews.
>
> 6. Blacks are twice as likely as whites to say that their health is poor and substantially less likely than whites to say that their health is good.
>
> 7. Blacks are twice as likely as whites to say that their health is worse than the health of other people their age.[20]

Although these findings have all of the limitations of self-reported survey data and cannot be assumed to reflect what would be found from physical examinations, this survey suggests that some of the physical difficulties that may lead to residence in a nursing home are more common among elderly blacks than among elderly whites. To the extent that poor health and the need for assistance in tasks of daily living define a need for nursing home care for non-institutionalized people, the need appears greater among the black elderly.

Among nursing home residents there is little racial difference in various measures of need and dependency. The 1977 National Nursing Home Survey found that black and white residents of nursing homes exhibit similar patterns of dependency in six activities of daily

Table 16. SELECTED MEASURES OF HEALTH LIMITATIONS AND DISABILITY FOR THE POPULATION 45+ YEARS OLD, BY RACE AND AGE (Data exclude persons in institutions)

Type of Limitation or Disability	45-64 years			65+ years		
	Black (%)	White (%)	Ratio: Black to White	Black (%)	White (%)	Ratio: Black to White
LIMITATION OF ACTIVITY, 1977[1]						
Total	100.0	100.0	1.00	100.0	100.0	1.00
Limited in activity	29.6	22.5	1.32	54.9	42.0	1.31
Limited in major activity	25.8	17.9	1.44	50.9	36.1	1.41
Limited in amount or kind of major activity	15.6	12.0	1.30	23.6	19.8	1.19
Unable to carry on major activity	10.1	5.9	1.71	27.3	16.3	1.67
Not limited in major activity	3.8	4.6	0.83	4.0	5.8	0.69
Not limited in activity	70.4	77.5	0.91	45.1	58.0	0.78
LIMITATIONS OF MOBILITY, 1972[1]						
Total	100.0[2]	100.0	1.00	100.0[2]	100.0	1.00
Limited in mobility	8.6	4.4	1.95	23.7	17.0	1.39
Has trouble getting around alone	4.3	2.2	1.95	7.7	5.6	1.38
Needs help in getting around	1.6	1.0	1.60	8.3	6.5	1.28
Not limited in mobility	91.4	95.6	0.96	76.3	83.0	0.92
DAYS OF RESTRICTED ACTIVITY, 1977						
Average number of days per year	35.5	23.1	1.54	59.6	36.4	1.64
DAYS OF BED DISABILITY, 1977						
Average number of days per year	13.9	7.9	1.76	24.6	11.7	2.10

[1]Data refer to limitations due to chronic conditions.
[2]Data on limitation of mobility are for all nonwhite races.

SOURCE: Administration on Aging, Characteristics of the Black Elderly--1980, DHEW Publication No. (OHDS) 80-20057 (Washington, D.C.: DHEW, 1980). The sources of the data are National Center for Health Statistics, Vital and Health Statistics, Series 10, No. 96, Limitation of Activity and Mobility due to Chronic Conditions: United States--1972; No. 126, Current Estimates from the Health Interview Survey: United States--1977; and unpublished data from the 1977 Health Interview Survey.

Table 17. PERCENT DISTRIBUTION OF NURSING HOME RESIDENTS BY DEPENDENCY IN ACTIVITIES OF DAILY LIVING, ACCORDING TO RACIAL OR ETHNIC STATUS OF RESIDENTS, 1977

Race or Ethnicity	All Residents	Dependency in Activities of Daily Living					
		Requires Assistance in Bathing	Requires Assistance in Dressing	Requires Assistance in Using Toilet Room	Mobility--Walks with Assistance or Is Chairfast or Bedfast	Continence--Difficulty with Bowel and/or Bladder Control	Requires Assistance in Eating
White (not Hispanic)	100.0	86.5	69.3	52.3	66.0	45.2	32.4
Black (not Hispanic)	100.0	85.7	73.9	55.7	67.0	48.5	34.0
Hispanic, American Indian, Alaska native, Asian or Pacific Islander	100.0	76.7	62.9	51.1	67.7	38.0	36.0

SOURCE: National Center for Health Statistics, Nursing Home Survey: 1977 Summary for the United States, (Washington, D.C.: Government Printing Office, 1979), p. 45.

living (Table 17).[21] The few differences show black nursing home residents to be slightly more dependent than whites. However, the racial differences in disability among nursing home residents are clearly smaller than such differences among the non-institutionalized population, which suggests that a smaller proportion of the disabled elderly black population than of the disabled elderly white population is admitted to nursing homes.

To summarize, evidence from national surveys shows that although disability is more common among elderly blacks than among elderly whites, use of nursing homes is substantially higher for whites than for blacks. The probability that a disabled, elderly black person will be admitted to a nursing home appears to be much lower than the probability that an elderly white person will be admitted. Two principal explanations have been offered for the low rates of nursing home use among blacks. The first pertains to values and living arrangements that characterize the black family. The second pertains to the availability of nursing home beds for blacks and involves geographic and economic factors and the possibility of racial discrimination.

Family Factors and Nursing Home Use

It is frequently suggested that the relatively low use of nursing homes by both black and Hispanic elderly is at least partially due to certain values and characteristics of families in these minority groups. Regarding values, it is pointed out that racial and ethnic groups differ about such matters as the esteem in which the elderly are held and the extent to which the elderly play an active role in family life. For example, the sociologist Robert Hill says of the black family:

> With respect to family composition, it is very important to note that elderly persons have been a major source of stability for black families from slavery to present times. In fact, it is the role of the elderly that is primarily responsible for the strong kinship bonds in most black families.[22]

Patterns of exchange that have been described in urban areas may facilitate the community care of persons who need assistance in managing some of the basic tasks of life. This is described (though not in relation to the elderly) in the summary of Carol Stack's rich ethnographic account of the black family in an urban neighborhood:

> Black families in The Flats and the non-kin they regard as kin have evolved patterns of co-residence, kinship-based exchange networks linking multiple domestic units, elastic household boundaries, lifelong bonds to three-generation households, social controls against the formation of marriages that could endanger the networks of kin, the

> domestic authority of women, and limitations on the role of the husband or male friend within a woman's kin network. These highly adaptive structural features of urban black families comprise a resilient response to the social-economic conditions of poverty, the inexorable unemployment of black women and men, and the access to scarce economic resources of a mother and her children as AFDC recipients.[23]

Wershow writes of a pilot study in Alabama in which he had expected to find elderly black women in non-institutional settings because of a child care role that they provided in their families. Instead, he found

> a number of elderly blacks, mostly females living in stable communities, were living at home because neighbors and church members helped in accordance with well organized plans. Most recipients of this neighborly aid have been pillars of the church and especially active in Ladies Missionary work, who are now reaping the fruits of their long years of faithful service by these church-organized volunteers.[24]

However, even if substantial resources of kin are available in neighborhoods, the needs for care and assistance that may develop in very old age may present very formidable demands. The evidence that values of mutual assistance play a substantial role in affecting black use of nursing homes is still scanty.

Differing values are not the only familial explanation that has been offered to account for racial/ethnic variations in nursing home use. The National Nursing Home Survey (1977) showed less than half (44 percent) of nursing home residents to be receiving "intensive" nursing care.[25] Such data often are cited to support the point that the use of nursing homes depends in part on the availability or non-availability of family members (usually the spouse or adult offspring) to provide care at home.[26] Thus, the living arrangements of elderly and disabled persons may play a significant role in their need for long-term care, particularly in intermediate care facilities, and it is suggested that certain living arrangements found more commonly among minority groups may well facilitate home care for dependent elderly people.

Without question, there are racial differences in the frequency with which certain living arrangements are found. Detailed data on the living arrangements of people aged 65 and older were collected in the 1968 Social Security Survey of the Demographic and Economic Characteristics of the Aged. Table 18 summarizes the data on race and living arrangements. Non-whites were less likely than whites to be living as married couples. However, white households (for both married couples and unmarried women) were much less likely than black households to include other relatives (most commonly children and grandchildren). The Census Bureau's Annual Housing Survey provides

Table 18. LIVING ARRANGEMENTS BY RACE: PERCENTAGE DISTRIBUTION OF AGED UNITS BY TYPE OF ARRANGEMENT, BY RACE OF UNIT, 1968

Type of Arrangement	Married Couples		Nonmarried persons: Men		Nonmarried persons: Women	
	White	Negro	White	Negro	White	Negro
Total Number (in thousands)	5,584	386	2,090	251	6,852	567
Total Percent	100	100	100	100	100	100
No relatives present	82	64	66	67	62	48
Alone	81	61	51	50	50	37
With nonrelatives	1	3	5	15	3	8
In institutions	*	*	10	2	8	3
Relatives Present	18	36	33	33	38	52
Children	14	20	21	18	28	33
Under age 18 only	1	3	*	2	*	
No children	4	16	12	14	10	19
Grandchildren	4	17	11	9	10	21
Brother or sister	1	1	9	8	8	9
Parents	*	*	*	2	*	*
Other relatives	4	11	17	15	16	22

*0.5 percent or less.

SOURCE: Janet Murray, "Living Arrangements of People Aged 65 and Older: Findings from the 1968 Survey of the Aged," Social Security Bulletin (September 1971) p. 7.

additional information on racial differences in living arrangements (Table 19). The black elderly are dispersed among a larger number of households, reflecting higher rates of separation and divorce. Thirty percent of black households include a person aged 65 and above, compared with 22 percent of white households and 16 percent of "Spanish origin" households. Almost all (95 percent) whites aged 65 and above live in households headed by a person aged 65 and above, while this is true for just over half (54 percent) of blacks. Finally, the Census Bureau's figures show that whites aged 65 and above are much more likely than either blacks or Spanish-origin persons to live alone.

The percentage of the black aged who share a household with their grown children is larger than for whites, but blacks are only slightly more likely than whites to live near their children. Thus, a national survey of the aged conducted in the mid-1970s found that the portion of old people whose nearest child is either in the same household or no more than 10 minutes away is 59 percent for blacks and 52 percent for whites.[27]

Table 19. HOUSING CHARACTERISTICS OF THE POPULATION AGED 65 AND OVER, BY RACE, 1977

	(A) Households (by Race of Head)	(B) Households Containing at Least One Person Aged 65 and Above	(B/A)	(C) Households Headed by Person Aged 65 and Above	(C/B)	(D) Households Containing One Person Aged 65 and Above Living Alone	(D/C)
Total	75,280,000	16,940,000	23%	15,035,000	89%	6,542,000	39%
White	63,710,000	14,043,000	22%	13,381,000	95%	5,850,000	42%
Black	7,956,000	2,389,000	30%	1,280,000	54%	559,000	23%
Spanish Origin	3,614,000	508,000	16%	374,000	74%	133,000	26%

SOURCE: Bureau of the Census, Annual Housing Survey, 1977, Part A, General Housing Characteristics (Series H-150-77).

Differences in living arrangements, however, do not necessarily imply differences in family resources available to the elderly. For example, in Shanas's national survey of the aged, there was virtually no difference between blacks (78 percent) and whites (76 percent) in reports of having visited with children during the previous week.[28] It appears that the racial difference in living arrangements may be an indicator more of economic or cultural differences rather than differences in the degree of social isolation of the elderly. Nevertheless, living arrangements that are found more often in the black family would appear to facilitate the home care of elderly persons who have become partially disabled.

Yet there is some evidence that there may not be racial differences in whether partially disabled, elderly people are able to obtain needed assistance within their homes. Shanas's survey of the black aged focused particularly on patterns of assistance for elderly persons with various types of disabilities.[29] The data are shown in Table 20. There was little overall racial difference in receipt of needed care from family members, although for whites this was more likely to come from a spouse (reflecting the racial difference in marital status) and blacks were more likely to be helped by relatives (other than children) living in or outside the household. Persons who had been "ill in bed" were asked about receipt of three types of help; whites were less likely to have received help in these circumstances. For persons needing three types of help (persons who were unable to care for their feet, persons unable to perform heavy household tasks, and persons having difficulty with meal preparation), blacks were slightly less likely than whites to have received help. Whites were more likely than blacks to have purchased help (from a podiatrist for foot care or a paid helper for household tasks). There was no consistent racial pattern in receiving help from unrelated persons outside of the household.

Similar findings come from a study of "functional social networks" of black, Hispanic, and white elderly persons in New York City.[30] Although there were differences among these groups regarding which sources of help were primary (for example, blacks were lowest in reliance on spouses, and Hispanics were notably high in the importance of children), those that mentioned no help sources were very few and were in roughly the same proportion among whites (6.6 percent), blacks (4.3 percent), and Hispanics (4.6 percent).

Although the data from the Shanas study show living arrangements to be reflected in the sources of assistance received by the elderly, neither of these studies shows an overall, consistent racial difference in the ability of the elderly to obtain needed help outside of a nursing home. This casts doubt on the hypothesis that blacks are not found in nursing homes because they are more able than whites to obtain needed care at home due to living arrangements that are more typical of the black family. Firm conclusions about the role of family factors and living arrangements in explaining racial/ethnic differences in the use of nursing homes must await the conduct of additional studies in which the living arrangements of patients (with specified levels of disability or with carefully defined needs for

Table 20. SOURCES OF CARE, FOR PERSONS AGED 65 AND OVER, BY RACE AND TYPE OF ASSISTANCE NEEDED, 1975 (Percent Using Source)

Type of Assistance	Spouse		Child in Household		Child Outside Household		Others in Household		Private Podiatrist		Paid Helper		Social Services		Relatives Outside Household		Non-relative Outside Household		None	
	White	Black	White	Black	White	Black	White	Black	White	Black	White	Black	White	Black	White	Black	White	Black	White	Black
Housework assistance for persons who had been ill in bed	38	32	13	11	14	14	3	13			9	4	0	2	4	7	2	9	24	15
Meal preparation for persons who had been ill in bed	41	33	11	12	14	15	4	14			3	2	1	1	4	7	6	15	25	16
Help with shopping for persons who had been ill in bed	39	33	14	13	20	17	4	12			2	2	0	*	6	8	13	10	13	9
Help for persons needing foot care	29	15	18	17	12	16	2	14	31	19			2	3	3	9	6	5	2	6
Help for persons needing help with heavy household tasks	26	21	16	13	15	14	4	16			29	12	1	0	4	10	2	4	10	20
Help for persons having difficulty with meal preparation	43	29	27	21	6	10	4	18			7	6	2	0	6	5	1	3	14	16

*Less than 1 percent after rounding.

SOURCE: Shanas, Ethel, National Survey of Black Aged, Final Report to Social Security Administration, no date.

assistance) from different racial/ethnic groups are compared and related to familial characteristics, socioeconomic factors, and the expressed preferences of patients and caregivers.

The role of values, family, and socioeconomic factors (for example, the resources to hire someone to provide assistance in the home) cannot now be distinguished from the role of the non-availability or the inaccessibility of nursing home facilities. Thus, even if it could be shown that elderly blacks with a given level of disability or need for assistance are more likely than elderly whites to stay with their families, the role of choice in this matter would remain unclear. That is, such a finding could be due to values or structural factors (such as multiple generations in the same household) that are more common in the black family, or it could be due to an attenuated range of options that may be available to many black families.

That familial and residential factors may not explain low black use of nursing homes is reinforced by data on overall patterns of institutionalization among black and white elderly populations. The 1970 census data show that only 56 percent of the institutionalized elderly non-whites were in "homes for the aged," compared with 80 percent of institutionalized elderly white persons, while elderly non-whites were markedly overrepresented in mental hospitals and chronic disease hospitals (such as TB).[31] The extent to which these trends reflect blocked access to nursing homes, rather than racial differences in health status, is unknown. Data on the extent of black residence in unlicensed boarding and personal care homes would also be instructive in evaluating the extent to which the low representation of blacks in nursing homes reflects blocked access.

Less information is available on the role of familial factors in affecting nursing home use of ethnic minorities other than blacks. A recent Federal Council on the Aging staff report on elderly minorities suggests that the "bond between the natural support networks and older persons" is undergoing more stress among Pacific Asians and Hispanics than among blacks.[32] However, little evidence was presented to show that this is true. The report also suggests that members of ethnic minorities may be particularly reluctant to use long-term care facilities, because of "fear of being removed from their cultural surroundings," and emphasizes the importance of cultural factors and language barriers in influencing ethnic minorities' ability to obtain needed services.[33] These factors may have particular force on the long-term care context (as opposed to acute hospitalization) because of its residential aspect.

Although the causal role of values and familial factors cannot now be assessed with certainty and may differ among various ethnic minorities, evidence examined by the committee suggests that, at least with regard to the black elderly, the most important factors underlying their low use of nursing homes pertain to the non-availability of beds. Beds may be unavailable either because they do not exist or because they are in some sense reserved for other people. Most nursing homes are private and can set their own rules for admission, such as an unwritten rule that you must be able to pay your own way for a year before going on Medicaid, with its lower reimbursement rates. The factors underlying the non-availability of beds and the reasons why this, rather than values or familial factors may best explain the low rates of nursing home use among blacks, are examined in the next section.

Factors Affecting the Availability of Nursing Homes for Minorities

A number of factors may result in restricted availability of beds to minority group members. These include location of nursing homes, patients' ability to pay for care, and racial discrimination.

Geographic Factors The location of nursing homes may negatively affect their use by minority groups in two ways. First, the lack of proximity of nursing homes to minority neighborhoods is a possible factor. Location near family is frequently a factor in selection of a nursing home.[34] The National Nursing Home Survey (1977) showed that almost two-thirds of nursing home residents had visitors on a daily or weekly basis, usually from relatives.[35] However, the committee did not locate any studies of the geographical patterns of nursing homes. However, given what is known about the availability of other types of medical care, it seems likely that nursing homes tend to be located away from predominantly black areas of cities. The same is probably true for the rural South.

Second, nursing home beds tend to be in shorter supply in states with relatively high proportions of blacks. Scanlon, Difederico, and Stassen suggest that at least part of the national racial difference in nursing home use may be accounted for by "the concentration of black elderly in low income states, particularly the Southeast," that may not be willing to support a large nursing home population with public funds.[36] About one-half of blacks in the United States reside in the South,[37] which is the region with the lowest rate of utilization of nursing homes. Approximately 2.6 percent of the population aged 65 and above in the South reside in nursing homes, compared with 5 percent in New England and 4 percent in the Pacific states.[38] The nature of any causal relationship between the concentration of blacks and the existence of nursing home beds is undoubtedly complex.

Financial Factors The association between race and income in the United States is well established.[39] Data from a recent national survey by the National Center for Health Statistics, for example, found family incomes of under $5,000 for 30 percent of blacks, 19 percent of Hispanics, 12 percent of Asian or Pacific Islanders, and 11 percent of whites.[40] The elderly black population is disproportionately dependent upon Medicaid for meeting the expenses of long-term care. The 1977 National Nursing Home Survey found that personal or family income was the primary source of support for 40.5 percent of white nursing home residents but for only 13 percent of black residents. Conversely, Medicaid was the primary source of support for 72.5 percent of black residents and for 46 percent of white residents.

Dependence on Medicaid has significant disadvantages for persons seeking nursing home care. In some states there have been serious delays in the process of making determinations of eligibility for Medicaid.[41] This may result in patients remaining in hospitals who could be cared for in nursing homes. More important, because the demand for nursing home care exceeds the supply of beds in many, perhaps most, locations and because three-fourths of nursing homes maintain a waiting list, nursing home operators often have the opportunity to choose between a Medicaid patient and a private-pay patient when a vacancy occurs.[42] Payment levels under Medicaid are controlled by each state and, because of cost-containment considerations, are generally lower than the rates charged by nursing homes to private-pay patients. The latter may eventually exhaust their resources and become Medicaid patients, but initially they can be expected to pay more than the Medicaid level. Indeed, the practice of charging non-publicly supported patients more than cost in order to make up for deficits resulting from low rates paid for publicly paid patients--cross-subsidization--is well known,[43] and it is often argued that a substantial representation of privately paying patients is essential to the viability of nursing homes. In Scanlon's words, "Cognizant of its oligopsony power as the largest purchaser of nursing home care, the government does not pay the market price. Instead, the state establishes a rate at which it will reimburse homes for care for an eligible person."[44] Rational economic behavior of nursing homes is to accept as many private patients as possible, even if some of them will eventually transfer to Medicaid.

An additional deterrent to the admission of Medicaid patients is the fact that their admission is accompanied by government-required review procedures designed to restrict unnecessary use of services. These procedures can put the Medicaid patient at a disadvantage compared with the private-pay patient who may be admitted without such review.[45] In addition to reimbursement rates that make Medicaid patients less attractive than private-pay patients, providers face more paperwork with the Medicaid patient and have complained in some states about delays in receiving payment under Medicaid.

These various circumstances appear to be reflected in behavior by providers that is not to the advantage of Medicaid patients. In the words of the New York State Moreland Act Commission, "the problem of discrimination against Medicaid-paid patients is apparent to virtually every knowledgeable person from whom the Commission has heard."[46] In the IOM committee's experience, knowledgeable people continue to express certainty that Medicaid patients are discriminated against by nursing homes because of the factors already mentioned. Scanlon, an economist, assumes that proprietary nursing homes "operate as profit maximizers" and therefore "will want to discriminate between private-pay and Medicaid residents."[47] He goes on to argue that non-profit nursing homes will behave similarly because of their own incentives to maximize income. The forms of discrimination that allegedly occur are not confined to a reluctance or refusal to admit Medicaid patients. There may also be refusals to admit private-pay patients who are likely to exhaust assets and go onto Medicaid relatively quickly, and there are allegations that nursing homes that do not accept Medicaid patients sometimes divest themselves of patients who are shifting to Medicaid payment. There is nothing to force a home that does not accept Medicaid patients to retain a patient whose private funds have been exhausted. Such patients must shift for themselves, joining the line of Medicaid patients waiting (often in hospitals) for available Medicaid space in a nursing home.

With the different levels of payment for nursing home care, economic discrimination against Medicaid patients is inevitable. Yet the situation and its differential effect on minority groups is not well documented. Records may be available through utilization review programs that would at least allow comparisons to be made among hospitalized patients in the amount of time spent awaiting nursing home placements. Such an approach was used in a recent study of the "hospital backup" problem of hospitalized patients awaiting placement in nursing homes, which was conducted by the Office of the Inspector General in DHHS Region 10.[48] Characteristics of such patients at a sample of 57 hospitals were collected. For 66 percent of these patients, Medicaid was to be the initial source of payment for their nursing home care (6 percent would be self-pay patients), and Medicaid was the likely eventual source of payment for 88 percent. By comparison, the 1977 National Nursing Home Survey found 38 percent of nursing home patients to be self-pay (including family payment) and 48 percent to be Medicaid patients. This 48 percent includes an unknown, but presumably large number of persons who began on other forms of payment and went onto Medicaid after their Medicare or private insurance benefits ran out or their assets had been depleted. (The proportion of nursing home patients who are on Medicaid at the outset must be considerably smaller than 48 percent.) Thus, the study suggests that Medicaid patients make up a disproportionately large share of the pool of hospitalized patients awaiting nursing home placement.

Virtually nothing is known about the characteristics of non-hospitalized persons who are seeking placement in a nursing home. A study of such persons would involve more primary data collection and some difficult sampling problems, but is necessary to a full understanding of the placement issue since placement from home involves different processes and actors than placement from a hospital.

Adequacy of These Explanations It is likely that the low use of nursing homes by blacks may be due, in part, to successful adaptations within families and neighborhoods, the disproportionate location of blacks in states where nursing homes are in short supply, and their relative poverty and disproportionate membership in a class--Medicaid patients--that is itself discriminated against. However, examination of patterns of nursing home use reveals a number of other aspects that cannot be readily explained in terms of these factors. Among these patterns are some large racial differentials among Medicaid patients, patterns of racial segregation among nursing homes in some locales, and variations from place to place in the extent of black use of nursing homes.

Racial Differentials in Medicaid One way to assess the role of economic factors in the lower black usage of nursing homes is to examine variations among persons who have a similar economic position and who are using the same source of payment for care. Racial differences within Medicaid, the largest single source of payment for nursing home care, could hardly be attributed to economic factors. Statistics published by the Health Care Financing Administration about the Medicaid program have been the source of much concern about inequity in the program. However, data problems similar to those discussed in Chapter 2--the absence of data regarding the population from whom Medicaid beneficiaries are drawn and failure of many states to report utilization statistics by race-- make it difficult to assess adequately the question of equity in nursing home expenditures under Medicaid.

For example, the DHEW publication, "Health Status of Minorities and Low-Income Groups," includes a chart showing the racial distribution of different types of services under Medicaid. The ratio of whites to non-whites (per 1,000 beneficiaries) is shown to be 3.23 for "nursing homes" and 4.01 for intermediate care facilities.[49] However, in the absence of data about either the characteristics of the pool from which beneficiaries are drawn or the age distributions of white and non-white Medicaid beneficiaries, interpretation of even such large apparent differences is speculative. The differences may be due, for example, to the greater frequency of the aged in the white Medicaid population. Nevertheless, these data are sometimes cited as evidence of racial inequity in nursing home care under Medicaid.

However, some less ambiguous Medicaid data suggest that problems of racial equity exist regarding nursing home care. Several states that have significantly large minority populations do report their Medicaid utilization data by race. Although these states cannot be assumed to represent the United States as a whole, it is, nevertheless, instructive to examine their racial patterns in use of long-term care facilities under Medicaid.

Data on racial patterns in Medicaid-paid nursing home use in this selected and diverse group of states is shown in Table 21. Data are presented separately for skilled nursing and intermediate care facilities; the fact that there are substantial variations among states in Medicaid benefits (particularly regarding skilled nursing) must be kept in mind because this greatly affects the absolute number of beneficiaries in various states. The available Medicaid data are provided for patients classified as white or "other," because they were collected on forms that offered only those choices. (This has undergone revision in accord with the more recent government-wide policy to standardize the collection of racial data.) For comparison, state data on the racial composition of the population above age 65 also are presented (more than 80 percent of nursing home residents are above age 65, according to the 1977 National Nursing Home Survey). Finally, data on the racial makeup of the poor population aged 65 and above in these states are presented and provide the most relevant point of comparison since this is the population from which the Medicaid-paid nursing home population is primarily drawn.

Table 21. BLACK/NONWHITES IN SELECTED STATES AS A PERCENT OF THE AGED POPULATION, THE AGED POOR POPULATION, AND MEDICAID RECIPIENTS FOR INTERMEDIATE CARE AND SKILLED NURSING FACILITIES

States	Percent of Population Age 65 and Above Who Are Black[1]	Percent of Poverty Population Age 65 and Above Who Are Black[2]	Non-white Medicaid Recipients, 1976[3]			
			Intermediate Care Facilities		Skilled Nursing Facilities	
			Number of Beneficiaries	Percent Non-white	Number of Beneficiaries	Percent Non-white
Alabama*	27.1	37.0	6,897	21.4	13,575	19.8
Arkansas	18.5	26.4	14,917	26.5	4,465	27.5
Delaware	11.0	18.7	1,133	48.0	107	76.0
Georgia*	21.2	29.5	13,433	31.0	4,246	22.0
Kansas	3.6	5.9	14,129	5.3	1,721	8.4
Kentucky	7.1	9.2	7,000	9.0	6,558	9.6
Maryland	13.5	24.6	7,225	16.3	1,948	24.8
Michigan	7.7	11.7	22,315	12.2	32,169	11.6
Minnesota**	0.5	0.6	24,669	1.5	19,297	1.6
Mississippi*	36.2	49.2	1,575	21.3	8,363	20.8
Missouri*	7.3	10.1	8,928	10.0	3,351	12.7
Nebraska	1.4	2.4	9,167	2.5	876	7.3

New Jersey*	6.2	11.1	22,878	12.9	3,007	13.0
Ohio*	6.7	10.8	16,916	12.5	25,884	14.5
Oklahoma	6.4	9.6	22,500	10.2	284	22.9
Oregon**	0.8	1.1	10,233	2.6	910	2.9
South Carolina*	28.4	43.0	3,602	34.5	7,491	36.1
Tennessee	15.0	20.3	17,019	20.4	600	46.3
Texas*	10.7	16.8	76,900	15.7	10,473	16.4
Virginia	17.9	28.3	12,033	24.8	1,372	35.0

*States that do not include medically needy under Medicaid (Janet B. Mitchell and Jerry Cromwell, Large Medicaid Practices: Are They Medicaid Mills? Health Care Financing Grants and Contracts Reports Series (Washington, D.C.: DHEW, 1980, p. 41).
**Under 1,000 blacks, 1965.

[1]SOURCE: U.S. Census, 1970.
[2]Derived from Bureau of the Census, General Social and Economic Characteristics, 1970 census
[3]SOURCE: Health Care Financing Administration, Medicaid State Tables, Fiscal Year 1976; Recipients, Payments and Services (Washington, D.C.: DHEW).

Table 21 shows that the black use of nursing homes under Medicaid is quite variable when considered against the racial makeup of the elderly poor population in the various states. For many states, the percentage of black Medicaid patients in nursing homes is quite similar to the percentage of blacks among the poor aged population. However, in a few states--most notably Alabama, South Carolina, and Mississippi--there are large differences. (There are a few counter-trends in a few other states where numbers are small.) In Mississippi, almost half of the elderly poor are black, but only about 20 percent of nursing home patients are black. In some states (for example, Maryland and Oklahoma) the racial composition of one type of nursing facility (skilled or intermediate care) reflects the characteristics of the poor aged of the state, while the other type of facility does not. This may be associated with state restrictions on benefits for one or the other type of nursing home, but it is not clear why the racial makeup of the two types of facilities differs.

While the data do not explain the reasons for the variations within and between states, Table 21 does illustrate several important points. First, aggregate data for some states show a pattern that strongly suggests racial inequity in long-term care under Medicaid. For some reason, poor white elderly patients in these states obtain nursing home care at much higher rates than do poor black elderly patients. Second, the data show that states are not uniform in this regard; nursing home benefits in many states are provided in rough proportion to the needy population in those states. Thus, the low rate of nursing home use by blacks must be due to factors that vary from state to state.

The fact that elderly black Medicaid patients in many states use nursing homes at roughly the same rate as elderly whites casts doubt on the suggestion that values and family structure generally underlie lower black use of nursing homes. Since it can be argued (based on the rates of disability and chronic illess among elderly blacks and whites) that use of nursing homes should be higher among blacks than among whites, it is still possible that familial factors have some effect on black use of nursing homes. However, since in many states the rates of nursing home use among poor blacks are as high as among poor whites, closer attention seems warranted in locales where blacks use nursing homes at substantially lower rates than do whites.

Urban Variations in Nursing Home Use Although comparisons among cities and states in the relationship of white to non-white use of nursing homes can facilitate the identification of possible reasons for the overall racial difference in use of nursing homes, few studies exist that describe the overall patterns of use within specific geographic areas. Systematic data do not exist on the extent of variation from city to city in minority group use of nursing homes, but studies in Baltimore and Philadelphia suggest that there may be great variation.

A study conducted in 1974 showed that the proportion of blacks in nursing homes both in Baltimore city and county exceeded the proportion of blacks in the 1970 census.[50] In Baltimore city, where blacks made up 25 percent of the population aged 65 and above, 32 percent of nursing home residents were black. By contrast, a study conducted in a similar city, Philadelphia, found that blacks made up only 13 percent of the nursing home population in 1978, compared with 20 percent of the population aged 65 and over in 1970.[51] (No similar racial discrepancy was found in two suburban counties in the Philadelphia study.) The racial difference between the two cities apparently is not due to gross differences in Medicaid eligibility standards. Both states include the medically needy in their Medicaid programs, and Pennsylvania actually includes a larger percentage of the poor under Medicaid than does Maryland.[52] It is unlikely that differences in values or family structures could account for such large differences in black nursing home use in the two cities. Thus, the explanation must be sought in such factors as racial attitudes, the supply of nursing home beds and their location, referral practices, and admission policies of nursing homes. Unfortunately, little information exists to enable the assessment of the way that these factors influence racial patterns in nursing home use in specific cities.

Racial Segregation in Nursing Homes If racial discrimination affects the use of nursing homes by minority groups, it is reasonable to expect this to be manifest not only in low nursing home use among minorities, but also in patterns of segregation. That is, if discrimination by some nursing homes underlies the disproportionately small numbers of elderly blacks in nursing homes, it would presumably also cause those blacks who are in nursing homes to be concentrated in a limited number of such facilities. Thus, in addition to racial segregation itself being a cause of concern in a multi-racial society, the extent of racial segregation may itself provide an indication that discrimination is taking place, even though other factors may also contribute to patterns of segregation. If the nursing homes tend to be segregated in the same cities or states where there is also notably low black usage of nursing homes, this could not be readily explained in terms of familial factors or values. The coincidence of patterns of low use and segregation is consistent with the hypothesis that racial discrimination is at work.

It is widely believed by persons familiar with nursing homes that they are characterized by a rather high degree of such segregation. Unfortunately, however, few data exist regarding the extent of racial segregation in nursing homes. There are historical reasons for concerns about segregation. Many facilities were established as private, non-profit institutions by religious or fraternal organizations (many of which are mono-racial) to take care of needy elderly members. Others grew out of the segregated "poor houses" of the South.

Some of the factors that lead to the concentration of certain ethnic groups in particular nursing homes are quite understandable--persons who do not speak English well are undoubtedly more comfortable and better off in a nursing home with others of their own culture than in a home where they are linguistically and culturally isolated. The same is true of persons who follow religiously imposed dietary restrictions. Nursing homes are in significant respects communities. It is not surprising that each seeks to create a harmonious group. However, such rationales also can be used to justify racial discrimination. As in other areas of our society, racial and ethnic patterns may develop both because persons of similar economic and cultural backgrounds tend to cluster and because persons of different backgrounds may be actively excluded. Self-exclusion by minority groups may occur as well, either by choice or because of fear of mistreatment or abuse in an alien ethnic setting. The role that these various considerations and processes play in the racial/ethnic sorting of nursing home residents has received little empirical study. The permissibility of these processes, particularly when tax dollars are paying for care, has yet to be fully addressed.

As in education, racial segregation in nursing homes may have an important impact on the resources available to the racial minorities. For example, in Kosberg's study of 214 nursing homes in the Chicago area, the adequacy of the treatment resources in facilities was negatively related to the percent of the facility's residents who were black. This largely reflected the resources that were available to the facility. Kosberg found a general pattern of few resources at institutions serving large numbers of poor (including black) patients because of the lower rates paid for their care. He also found that some nursing homes "managed to be rich in treatment resources" even though they had "sizable proportions of public aid recipients." These homes, he found, had raised the rates for private patients to make up for the money lost on public patients whose rates were below cost.[53]

Although there are obvious reasons for concern about racially segregated nursing homes, the matter has received little attention. The National Nursing Home Survey, conducted periodically by the National Center for Health Statistics, has not collected data that would allow measures, such as percentage of white patients, to be calculated for the separate nursing homes in the sample. The Nursing Home Survey's national estimates of minority group use of nursing homes are projected from data collected on the racial (and other) characteristics of only five sample patients per nursing home in the sample; thus, the data cannot be used as indicators of the racial composition of individual nursing homes and the extent to which minority group members are concentrated in a few nursing homes.

The Census Bureau's 1976 Survey of Institutionalized Persons may have obtained data that could be used to examine the extent of racial concentration in nursing homes.[54] Racial data were collected in interviews with residents of nursing homes; the sample was designed to include 10 residents in small institutions, 15 residents in medium-sized institutions, and numbers ranging from 15 to 40 in large institutions (where, incidently, blacks are disproportionately located according to the National Nursing Home Survey). However, no data have been published that show the degree of racial homogeneity or heterogeneity among residents (or staff members) of nursing homes.

Despite the absence of national data on racial clustering in nursing homes, there are indications that it is common. Some studies, focused on other issues, simply take racial segregation as a given. Wershow's study of black and white nursing home residents in Birmingham and rural Alabama provides an example. In describing his sampling approach, he refers to the seven "predominantly black nursing homes" in the state and to their white counterparts. He indicates that the few whites in the black nursing homes are the "most isolated of the long-term state mental hospital 'discharges to the community' who seem to have been selected as the first white nursing home patients to 'break the ice' of racial desegregation in the predominantly black nursing homes."[55] No information is provided about the number or characteristics of the black patients in the white nursing homes. Similarly, in her study of nursing home use in two East Coast cities, Schafft reported that there "remain racially identifiable hospitals and nursing homes. Repondents in the study referred to these institutions as 'black' and 'white'."[56] Schafft indicates that, although she has wanted to study racially integrated nursing homes, she has found almost none in four cities with which she has become familiar--Atlanta, Georgia; Washington, D.C.; Wilmington, Delaware; and Richmond, Virginia.[57]

Some scattered data are available about racial segregation in nursing homes. Race and admissions in 1978 to 133 nursing homes in Philadelphia, Montgomery, and Delaware counties in Pennsylvania were studied by two law students using records kept by the Pennsylvania Department of Health.[58] In all three counties, blacks tended to be concentrated in certain institutions. For example, there were fewer than 3 black patients in 36 of the 62 nursing homes in Philadelphia County (there were no blacks in 18 of these homes); 95 percent of the black residents were in the remaining (45 percent) nursing homes. Blacks were particularly overrepresented in black-owned and in public and hospital-affiliated homes. Blacks were virtually absent from non-profit homes in Montgomery and Delaware counties.

Data from the Baltimore study, though not presented in a way that allows for precise comparison with Philadelphia, suggest that a significant degree of racial clustering exists in Baltimore, although apparently less than in Philadelphia.[59] (Data are not presented that would enable the calculation of quantified indices of segregation for more precise comparisons of degree of segregation. Such an index could be based on the average variation from the overall mean number of white or non-white residents.*) However, of the approximately 45 nursing homes in Baltimore city, 4 had no minority patients, and 7-10 others had very few; at the other end of the scale, 9 facilities had more than 50 percent minority patients.

Apparently no other studies describe the degree of racial concentration in nursing homes or empirically explain patterns of racial clustering in nursing homes. The process by which persons and

---

*One measure that has been used in several studies is the Index of Dissimilarity, which is defined as one-half the sum of the absolute differences between two percentage distributions.[60]

nursing homes select each other (and the degree to which, and circumstances under which, residents choose which nursing home they will use, as opposed to taking what is available) has received little study. Little is known about matters such as the extent to which patterns of ownership and location may explain patterns of nursing home use, the extent to which the location of minority nursing home residents represents their (or their family's) choice, and the factors that may influence that choice (including the range of options and information available).

Racial Discrimination as an Explanation Most persons who have studied and written about black use of nursing homes believe that racial discrimination is a major explanatory factor for many of the racial patterns that have been described thus far. Testimony received by the committee strongly supports that point.[61] Because of both the history of racial discrimination in the United States and factors related to the origins and ownership of particular institutions, the likelihood that racial discrimination exists approaches certainty.

Racial discrimination is notoriously difficult to study directly (except in its most blatant forms) because it is usually not publicly acknowledged. The consequences of systematic discrimination, however, may show up in patterns such as have been described in this chapter--different rates of use of services, patterns of segregation, and so forth. Alternative explanations of racial patterns of nursing home use--demographic differences, differences in family values and living arrangements, and geographic and economic factors--appear to be inadequate to account for all the racial differences in nursing home use.

If, as the committee believes, racial discrimination affects nursing home use, it is important to identify ways in which it may operate and to suggest some potentially useful lines of research.

Discrimination may occur at many levels. At the federal and state levels, reimbursement practices reduce incentives to provide care for Medicaid patients, a population that is disproportionately made up of minority group members. State decisions on Medicaid coverage (for example, regarding inclusion of the "medically needy") have a strong effect on the ability of minority persons to obtain nursing home care. Recent analyses by economists suggest that governmental policies regarding the regulation of the bed supply in nursing homes may also work to the disadvantage of patients most in need of care.[62]

Discrimination can occur at many points in the process by which persons are referred to and gain admission to nursing homes. Many nursing home admissions are arranged by discharge planners in hospitals, and decisions are made that match patients and facilities. Very little systematic information exists about the criteria and the practices used, such as racial "steering," in referral. Many admissions are arranged through relationships established between particular hospitals and particular facilities. Schafft noted that in the two cities she studied, racially identified hospitals remain, and "doctors who practice in the 'black' institutions and those who practice in the 'white' institutions rarely cross over in placing their patients in nursing homes."[63] Because of racial patterning in the use of hospitals, nursing homes can influence the characteristics of the persons who are referred through the choice of hospitals with which relationships are established. The source of referrals can narrow the population from which a nursing home is drawing. If nursing home vacancies were filled through a central registry, the opportunity for homes to exercise racial criteria in admission would be greatly reduced. The example of one city cited by Schafft suggests that a central registry of vacancies in nursing homes may have a significant impact on the racial patterning in nursing homes.[64]

In sum, it appears that nursing homes have some ability to control the characteristics of patients referred. The range and type of sources from which a nursing home accepts referrals can heavily influence the characteristics of those who seek admission, and admissions criteria (for example, with regard to Medicaid patients) of nursing homes may have the practical effect of limiting the access of minority groups.

Many of these mechanisms are alleged to have been in play in Shelby County, Tennessee, according to litigation (Hickman v. Fowinkle, C.A. No. 80-2014, W.D. Tenn.) initiated in January 1980. There it is alleged that blacks are effectively denied admission to licensed, Medicaid-approved nursing homes and are relegated instead to unlicensed and unregulated boarding homes that do not provide the needed level of care. A number of practices are alleged to be involved, including giving preferential treatment to whites in admissions procedures, denying admission to applicants whose physicians do not have staff privileges at certain hospitals, and refusing to accept referrals from the county Department of Human Services.[65] The evidence developed in connection with these allegations may help to illuminate some practices that tend to maintain racially distinct patterns, as well as to determine the legal acceptability of such practices.

RESEARCH NEEDS

More certainty about the influence of various factors on the use of nursing homes could be gained through the collection of additional data on a routine or sample basis. Priority should be given to the conduct of studies to better document (a) the extent to which race or ethnicity influences whether persons who need the services of nursing homes are able to obtain such care and (b) the extent of racial segregation in nursing homes and the processes that contribute to it.

A variety of methods may prove useful in better documenting the characteristics and circumstances of partially disabled persons who do not reside in nursing homes. On the basis of census data and Medicare and Medicaid data, cities and states should be identified in which elderly persons from minority groups have a lower use of nursing homes. Efforts should be made to determine if race or ethnicity influence whether persons who need nursing home care are able to obtain it. In some instances, information about persons who are awaiting placement in nursing homes may be available from hospitals, professional standards review organizations (PSROs), or local social service agencies. However, because little information is available about what happens to people who need nursing home care but are unable to gain admission, empirical research should be conducted to increase our understanding of how people cope with this situation. One useful model is provided by Shanas's Survey of the Black Aged (cited in this chapter), which provided information about the sources of assistance used by aged persons living outside of institutionalized settings.

Better information is also needed about residents of unlicensed boarding homes, a population about which very little is known. It may be possible to sample such people by using addresses to which several Social Security checks are mailed (perhaps to persons who do not share a last name).

There is also a particular need for more systematic information about the extent to which nursing homes are racially segregated. The possibility that widespread patterns of discrimination exist in nursing home admissions has received little attention, either as a topic for research or as an object of civil rights enforcement activities. Such information probably can be developed by making use of data that are already being collected for other purposes. Racial/ethnic information on Medicare or Medicaid claims and eligibility files provide a basis for describing the extent to which the racial characteristics of nursing homes in any locale depart from the overall racial/ethnic composition of the elderly in that locale. That is, do the nursing homes in a locale all have approximately the same racial/ethnic composition (and, if so, does this roughly parallel the racial/ethnic composition of the elderly population of the locale), or do the nursing homes tend to be mostly white or black? In locales where the nursing homes tend toward segregation, research is needed on the process by which people enter a nursing home. For patients (or families) who selected a nursing home, how did they do so? Do they believe they encountered discrimination? Other patients reach nursing homes through referral processes about which they may know very little. Better information about the operation of such referral processes is needed. What arrangements exist between institutions (such as particular hospitals and particular nursing homes)? To what extent can nursing homes control the characteristics of patients through the referral networks that they establish? To what extent do hospital discharge planners consider racial/ethnic factors in making referrals and how aware are they of informal policies of discrimination practiced by nursing homes?

One source of information about racial/ethnic patterns in nursing homes is the data collected in connection with the annual certification procedures for nursing homes participating in Medicare and Medicaid. State certification teams are required by federal law (under guidelines issued in 1969) to conduct Title VI compliance review activities that include a one-day census of the race/ethnicity of patient populations. Although many (perhaps most) states apparently engage in such activities, little is known about how these censuses are used, whether the data in any states have ever been compiled so as to illuminate racial/ethnic patterns in the use of nursing homes, or whether the information has been used successfully in civil rights enforcement activities. Thus, a potentially useful source of information about the characteristics of nursing home residents may be readily available, at least in some states.

CONCLUSIONS

This chapter has reviewed evidence pertaining to the question of racial disparities in nursing homes. While the chapter demonstrates the difficulty of disentangling the possible causes of such disparities in nursing homes, the evidence suggests that discrimination may well be a factor in nursing home admissions. Research approaches are available that would help to further clarify the reasons underlying the racial patterns in nursing home use and the mechanisms that produce racial disparities. However, only if racial differences are seen as deserving serious attention can we come to understand adequately the impact of institutionalized mechanisms that lead to racial disparities in the American health care system.

REFERENCES

1. National Center for Health Statistics, The National Nursing Home Survey: 1977 Summary for the United States, Vital and Health Statistics, Series 13, No. 43, (Washington, D.C.: Government Printing Office, 1979) pp. 209-210.
2. Ibid., p. 8.
3. Ibid.
4. Bruce C. Vladeck, Unloving Care: The Nursing Home Tragedy (New York: Basic Books, 1980) p. 3.
5. The National Nursing Home Survey: 1977.
6. American Health Care Association, Long Term Care Facts (Washington, D.C.: AHCA, 1975) p. 7.
7. Congressional Budget Office, Long Term Care for the Elderly and Disabled (Washington, D.C.: Government Printing Office, 1977); United States Senate, Development in Aging: 1979, A Report of the Special Committee on Aging (Washington, D.C.: Government Printing Office, 1980).
8. Elaine Brody, "Environmental Factors in Dependency," in A. N. Exton-Smith and J. Grimley Evans (eds.), Care of the Elderly: Meeting the Challenge of Dependency (New York: Academic Press, 1977) p. 91.
9. Vladeck, p. 16.

10. William J. Scanlon, "A Theory of the Nursing Home Market," Inquiry 17 (Spring 1980) pp. 25-41.
11. Robert M. Gibson, "National Health Expenditures, 1978," Health Care Financing Review (Summer 1979) p. 26.
12. Scanlon, p. 25.
13. United States Senate, Trends in Long Term Care, Hearings Before the Subcommittee on Long-Term Care of the Special Committee on Aging, August 10, 1972, (Washington, D.C.: Government Printing Office, 1973) p. 2439.
14. National Center for Health Statistics, Characteristics of Residents in Nursing Homes and Personal Care Homes for U.S. June-August 1969, Vital and Health Statistics Series 12, No. 19 (Washington, D.C.: Government Printing Office, 1973) p. 2.
15. National Center for Health Statistics, Characteristics, Social Contacts, and Activities of Nursing Home Residents for U.S., 1973-1976, Vital and Health Statistics Series 13, No. 27 (Washington, D.C.: Government Printing Office, 1977) p. 3.
16. The National Nursing Home Survey: 1977, p. 29.
17. Characteristics, Social Contacts, and Activities of Nursing Home Residents, p. 6.
18. Department of Health, Education, and Welfare, Health United States: 1979 DHEW Publication No. (PHS) 80-1232 (Washington, D.C.: Government Printing Office, 1980) pp. 440-443.
19. Blanch Spruiel Williams, Characteristics of the Black Elderly, No. 5 in the Administration on Aging series of Statistical Reports on Older Americans (Washington, D.C.: DHHS, 1980) p. 40.
20. Ethel Shanas, "National Survey of the Aged: Final Report," Unpublished report on Social Security Administration Project Number 10 P - 57823, (no date) p. 5.
21. The National Nursing Home Survey: 1977, p. 45.
22. Jacqueline J. Jackson (ed.), Proceedings: Research Conference on Minority Group Aged in the South (Durham, NC: Duke University Medical Center, Center for Study of Aging and Human Development, 1972).
23. Carol B. Stack, All Our Kin: Strategies for Survival in a Black Community (New York: Harper and Row, 1974) p. 124.
24. Harold J. Wershow, "A Pilot Study Comparing Certain Characteristics of Black and White Nursing Home Patients in Birmingham and Rural Alabama," Report to Administration on Aging, Department of Health, Education, and Welfare (Grant 93p-5734/04-01), (no date) p. 9.
25. The National Nursing Home Survey: 1977, p. 53.
26. William J. Scanlon, Elaine Difederico, and Margaret Stassen, Long-Term Care: A Current Experience and a Framework for Analysis (Washington, D.C.: The Urban Institute, 1979) p. 24.
27. Shanas, p. 16.
28. Ibid., p. 17.
29. Ibid.
30. Marjorie H. Cantor, "The Informal Support System of New York's Inner City Elderly: Is Ethnicity a Factor?" in Donald F. Gelfand and Alfred J. Kutzik (eds.), Ethnicity and Aging: Theory, Research, and Policy (New York: Springer, 1979).

31. Beth Soldo, "Accounting for Racial Differences in Institutionalized Placements," presented at the Annual Meeting of The Gerontological Society, November 1977.
32. Federal Council on the Aging, Policy Issues Concerning the Elderly Minorities: A Staff Report, Publication No. (OHDS) 80-20670, (Washington, D.C.: DHHS, 1980) p. 40.
33. Ibid.
34. Ethel Shanas, Personal Communication, August 5, 1980.
35. The National Nursing Home Survey: 1977, p. 59.
36. Scanlon, Difederico, and Stassen, p. 27.
37. Bureau of the Census, 1976 Survey of Institutionalized Persons: A Study of Persons Receiving Long Term Care, Current Population Reports, Special Studies, Series P-23, No. 69 (Washington, D.C.: Government Printing Office, 1978) p. 13.
38. Scanlon, Difederico, and Stassen, p. 30.
39. Bureau of the Census, pp. 19-59.
40. Health United States: 1979, p. 7.
41. New York Statewide Professional Standards Review Council, Inc., "Quarter-Billion Dollars in Medicare and Medicaid Money Wasted in New York State on Hospital Patients Awaiting Move to Nursing Homes," press release, May 20, 1980.
42. Scanlon; The National Nursing Home Survey: 1977, p. 13.
43. Jordan I. Kosberg, "Differences in Proprietary Institutions Caring for Affluent and Nonaffluent Elderly," The Gerontologist (Autumn 1973) p. 303.
44. Scanlon, p. 28.
45. New York State Moreland Act Commission, p. 8.
46. Ibid., p. 5.
47. Scanlon, p. 28.
48. Office of the Inspector General, Department of Health and Human Services, "Restricted Patient Admittance to Nursing Homes: An Assessment of Hospital Back Up. Draft Technical Report," July 1980.
49. Health United States: 1979, p. 264.
50. Office for Civil Rights, "Baltimore City and Baltimore County Nursing Home Referral Study," Unpublished report (DHEW, OCR, Region 3, 1974).
51. Vanessa J. Lawrence and Jill Duson Mirach, "Racial Discrimination in Nursing Home Admissions in the Greater Philadelphia Area," Health Law Project Library Bulletin IV (January 1979) pp. 20-27.
52. Janet B. Mitchell and Jerry Cromwell, Large Medicaid Practices: Are They Medicaid Mills? Health Care Financing Grants and Contracts Reports series, (Baltimore, MD: Health Care Financing Administration, 1980) p. 14.
53. Kosberg, p. 303.
54. Bureau of the Census, p. 363.
55. Wershow, p. 5.
56. Gretchen Schafft, "Nursing Homes and the Black Elderly: Utilization and Satisfaction," Proceedings of the Fifth North American Symposium on Long-Term Care Administration (Bethesda,

MD: American College of Nursing Home Administration, 1980) p. 106.

57. Gretchen Schafft, personal communication.
58. Lawrence and Mirach.
59. Office for Civil Rights, pp. 8-9.
60. Cary S. Kart and Barry L. Beckham, "Black-White Differentials in the Institutionalization of the Elderly: A Temporal Analysis," Social Forces 54 (June 1976) pp. 901-910.
61. Schafft; Susan Conner (National Citizens Coalition of Nursing Home Reform), Testimony before IOM Committee, Washington, D.C., June 6, 1980.
62. Judith Feder and William Scanlon, "The Shortage of Nursing Home Beds," Journal of Health Politics, Policy and Law 4 (Winter 1980).
63. Schafft, p. 106.
64. Ibid.
65. National Senior Citizens Law Center, "Race Discrimination in Nursing Homes," NSCLC Washington Weekly 4 (June 27, 1980) p. 6.

4

HEALTH CARE OF HANDICAPPED PERSONS

"No otherwise qualified handicapped individual in the United States . . . shall, solely by reason of his handicap, be excluded from the participation in, be denied the benefits of, or be subjected to discrimination under any program or activity receiving Federal financial assistance."[1]

The prohibition against discrimination that Congress put into Section 504 of the Rehabilitation Act of 1973, as amended, reflects both the right of handicapped persons to function as integral members of society and greater public awareness of the problems that they encounter. The passage of a law, however, does not produce an automatic change in social conditions or in public perceptions and behavior. This chapter provides a brief examination of problems in the health care of handicapped persons in light of their explicit coverage by anti-discrimination legislation.

As amended, the Rehabilitation Act defines as handicapped any person who has a physical or mental impairment that substantially limits one or more of the major activities of life, such as caring for one's self, performing manual tasks, walking, seeing, hearing, speaking, breathing, learning, and working. The act also covers persons who have a record of such an impairment or who are "regarded as having" such an impairment.[2] The breadth and non-specific nature of this definition cause problems in implementing the legislation, some of which are discussed in this chapter. Nevertheless, the legislative definition is used in this report.

The population encompassed by the act's definition is large and diverse. (For example, the regulations mention the following categories: orthopedic, visual, speech, and hearing impairments, cerebral palsy, epilepsy, muscular dystrophy, multiple sclerosis, cancer, heart disease, diabetes, mental retardation, emotional illness, drug addiction, and alcoholism.) Included are persons with permanent disabilities, such as blindness, that may prevent their full and active functioning in many activities, persons with chronic conditions for which relatively close medical management is essential, persons with severe injuries who may require long periods of rehabilitation, mentally retarded persons, and persons with chronic psychiatric problems. The health care needs of these persons are equally diverse. Some such needs are unique to persons with particular handicapping conditions. Some other needs of handicapped persons are similar to those of the general population, although some such needs can best be met by specialized personnel or in specialized facilities. Only in the most abstract sense can the single adjective "handicapped" describe such a diverse population.

Deterrents to suitable health care for the handicapped include a lack of personnel trained to communicate with deaf persons, architectural barriers, policies designed to exclude persons who are regarded as potentially heavy users of services from nursing homes and health maintenance organizations, financial and regulatory barriers built into federal and state programs (including programs that have been developed to meet needs of handicapped persons), shortages in personnel and facilities to deal with certain types of disabilities and chronic conditions, and shortcomings in attitudes and knowledge among health care workers. Some of the most important deterrents (financial, resource scarcity, and attitudes) call for remedies beyond the reach of Section 504's prohibitions on discrimination. Others are addressed in the regulations implementing Section 504, although little information exists regarding the impact of the regulations.

The Office for Civil Rights (OCR) in the Department of Health and Human Services (DHHS) is responsible for the enforcement of Section 504. Regulations implementing Section 504 were issued by the Department of Health, Education, and Welfare (DHEW) on May 4, 1977, and include sections on employment practices; program accessibility; preschool, elementary, secondary, and postsecondary education; and health, welfare, and other social services programs. Subpart F of the regulations states that health, welfare, and other social service programs, activities, and providers who receive or benefit from federal financial assistance may not:

- deny a qualifed handicapped person these benefits or services; [A "qualified" handicapped person is defined as one who meets the essential eligibility requirements for the receipt of such services.]
- afford a qualified handicapped person an opportunity to receive benefits or services that is not equal to that offered nonhandicapped persons;
- provide a qualified handicapped person with benefits or services that are not as effective as the benefits or services provided to others; [Benefits or services, to be "equally effective," need not produce the "identical result or level of achievement for handicapped persons, but must afford handicapped persons equal opportunity to obtain the same result, to gain the same benefits, or to reach the same level of achievement in the most integrated setting appropriate to the person's needs."]
- provide benefits or services in a manner that limits or has the effect of limiting the participation of qualified handicapped persons; or

• provide different or separate benefits or services to handicapped persons except where necessary to provide qualified handicapped persons with benefits and services that are as effective as those provided to others.[3]

The regulations also require that hospital emergency rooms provide auxiliary aids if necessary for persons with impaired sensory, manual, or speaking skills and that drug addicts and alcoholics receive non-discriminatory health services.

The usefulness of Section 504 in handling many problems is uncertain. In theory, Section 504 guarantees handicapped persons access and entitlement to federally assisted health programs equal to that of other members of the population. However, such a guarantee raises many issues that are not yet fully resolved. Such regulatory terms as "equal," "effective," and "necessary" have not been conceptualized in a manner that can be easily applied in research or in civil rights compliance activities. Furthermore, shortcomings in information for comparison with non-handicapped persons make it difficult to identify differential treatment and, when identified, to determine whether it is inconsistent with Section 504. It is not yet clear when, where, to whom, and to what the discrimination prohibition applies, and the substantive meaning of discrimination in a wide variety of specific contexts is yet to be specified.

The committee found little evidence of a consensus about the problems in health care that properly can be called discrimination against handicapped persons. For example, the regulations call for specific actions by health care providers based upon explicit attention to handicapping conditions, such as having interpreters or other aids available to communicate with deaf persons. To behave differently toward a person because of some characteristic of that person is to engage in behavior that fits a commonplace conception of discrimination. However, the behavior that is encouraged by the regulation is intended to operate for the benefit of the persons whose particular needs are being recognized. As such it is quite consistent with the basic ethos of medicine that emphasizes attention to the particular needs of particular patients.

ISSUES OF DEFINITION AND CONCEPT

Several problems of terminology should be acknowledged in a chapter about health care problems of handicapped person. First, a term such as "handicap" means more than an objective reality, such as the medical and functional characteristics cited earlier in the Section 504 definition.* The term also carries "emotional and cognitive

---

*The regulations implementing Section 504 define "physical or mental impairment" as (a) any physiological disorder or condition, cosmetic disfigurement, or anatomical loss affecting one or more of the

baggage" that may affect the behavior of both the person with the handicap and other members of the population.[4] One word--handicap--covers conditions as diverse as deafness, chronic depression, and paraplegia, and yet that word lends itself to a stereotype.

Some observers, for example, have noted that some persons respond to a particular impairment as if it were a general impairment, as when people raise their voices when speaking to a blind person, address questions to relatives that handicapped patients could easily answer, or ignore the handicapped person's own expertise in managing life with the handicap. To increase awareness of the consequences of the use of labels, some commentators draw distinctions between such concepts as handicap and disability and call attention to the extent to which limitations are the result of societal responses rather than physiological conditions.[6] While authors may differ in how they make this distinction, their point is that the degree of disability associated with a condition depends not only on the condition itself but also on the relationship between affected persons and their environment. Caution is required to avoid overgeneralized assumptions of the limitations that may be implied by such labels as handicapped or disabled.

An additional problem of definition stems from the fact that a variety of related terms--handicapped, disabled, impaired--are used with reference to the same population or segments thereof. The Section 504 definition of handicapped reflects its purpose to prohibit discrimination on a particular basis. Other statutory definitions reflect the needs of programs, for example, to define beneficiaries of various programs. In 1978, at least 66 programs (using 16 different definitions of "handicapped" or "disabled") in the DHEW existed for populations to which Section 504 also applies.[7] For example, the Social Security Act defines those eligible for "disability" insurance; Title V of the Public Health Service Act establishes diagnostic and treatment services for children who are "crippled"; the Rehabilitation, Comprehensive Services and Developmental Disabilities Amendments of 1978 provide specific programs and benefits to those who are "developmentally disabled." Although some of the same people may be included under numerous definitions, it is apparent that definitions can affect the availability of certain benefits for some groups or individuals.[8]

Differences in definitions create serious problems in data collection and in program management. Data from different programs

---

following body systems: neurological; musculo-skeletal; special sense organs; respiratory, including speech organs; cardiovascular; reproductive; digestive; genito-urinary; hemic and lymphatic; skin; and endocrine or (b) any mental or psychological disorder, such as mental retardation, organic brain syndrome, emotional or mental illness, and specific learning disabilities.[5]

are frequently hard to compare, causing difficulties in determining how many people are handicapped or disabled and what services they receive. In addition, operational definitions in surveys of handicapped persons must inevitably depart from the Section 504 definition, which defines handicap in terms of an impairment "that substantially limits one or more major life activities," a record of such an impairment, or being regarded as having such an impairment. Although such a definition may be appropriate to addressing the problem of discrimination related to a handicap, the definition is too vague for research and program management purposes. It would be difficult to enumerate people who have a record of such an impairment and probably would be impossible to enumerate people who "are regarded" (by whom?) as having such an impairment.

The Section 504 definition does not clearly differentiate handicapped persons (who may or may not have a disease or illness) from people with diseases or illnesses. This is a source of confusion about such matters as what problems are peculiar to handicapped people and what problems pertain to patients in general. This confusion also complicates the collection of relevant data. The research use of the Section 504 definition, as it now stands, probably would result in the inclusion of persons whose life activities were limited temporarily because of acute conditions. In addition, almost all conditions listed in the Section 504 definition are present to some degree in many people who are not regarded by themselves or by others as handicapped, although such conditions may cause them varying degrees of difficulty in performing "major life activities." Although Section 504 prohibits discrimination because of any such condition, it would be difficult to attempt to count all such people in any survey that is trying to enumerate the disabled or handicapped persons in a population.

Any good survey must have clear operational definitions about such matters as who is to be included within the boundaries of the survey; in surveys relevant to the concerns of this chapter such definitions are most commonly stated in terms of ability to fulfill various types of roles, such as work. However, the question of whether one is able to work is not the same as the question of whether one falls within the Section 504 definition of handicapped, because, for example, many people who work also have an "impairment that affects a major life activity." Thus, it probably is inevitable that the population about which data exist will never coincide completely with the population against whom discrimination is prohibited by Section 504. This problem bears scrutiny by those concerned with issues of parity and discrimination toward handicapped persons, including the OCR. Operational definitions of handicapping conditions are clearly feasible. Legal tests may lead to clearer specifications.

SIZE AND DEMOGRAPHIC CHARACTERISTICS OF THE HANDICAPPED POPULATION

Three general observations can be made about the population of handicapped and disabled persons in the United States. First, it is a significant proportion of the U.S. population. Second, handicapped persons are found in disproportionate numbers among the elderly, the poor, and minorities. Thus, they are vulnerable to a variety of forms of discrimination that their disabilities can heighten. They also are likely to require governmental support to meet their health care and other needs. Third, many serious problems characterize the statistics about this population. A recent review properly describes the data as "scattered, confused, and confusing."[9]

Estimates of the number of handicapped persons vary greatly, primarily because agencies or organizations collecting the data use different methods of gathering information and different terms to define the population. At the federal level, for example, data are collected on "impairments" and "chronic activity limitations" by the National Center for Health Statistics, but the Bureau of the Census and the Social Security Administration (SSA) collect information on "disability."* (The one ongoing enumeration of the total population is the U.S. Census, which decided against including questions regarding handicaps in the 1980 census. Thus the opportunity to collect data on all handicapped persons was lost until 1990.) For the most part, these surveys sample different populations in different years, exclude the institutionalized population, and are usually based on respondents' reports of their own status. Such methods have important limitations. For example, whether persons perceive themselves as disabled undoubtedly depends upon a variety of factors in addition to their "objective" condition; it may be influenced, for example, by the way that they have been defined and treated by others and by the nature of their work. Some conditions may be underreported in household surveys because of shame or embarrassment.

The most comprehensive and current data on disability come from the Health Interview Survey conducted by the National Center for Health Statistics in 1977. The data on seven common "impairments" are listed in Table 22. Although the table does not include mentally ill or mentally retarded persons, and includes an unknown proportion of persons with a variety of chronic conditions, the number of impairments listed in Table 22 totals more than 41 million. The number of persons who reported more than one impairment is not known.

---

*The most recent available SSA data are from the 1972 survey of disabled and non-disabled adults. Because the data are old, they are not reported here. In general, however, they are consistent with the general characteristics of the disabled that are described here.[10] Data from a 1978 survey of disabled adults by the Social Security Administration are not yet available, but are confined to persons with work disability.

Table 22. ESTIMATES OF PERSONS WITH SELECTED IMPAIRMENTS BY AGE AND SEX: UNITED STATES, 1977 (in thousands)

Type Impairment by Sex	Total	Age			
		17	17-44	45-64	65+
Blind and Visually Impaired					
Total	11,415	678	2,877	2,959	4,902
Male	5,910	436	1,891	1,702	1,881
Female	5,505	241	986	1,257	3,021
Deaf and Hearing Impaired					
Total	16,219	856	3,480	5,365	6,518
Male	8,925	489	2,093	3,233	3,110
Female	7,924	366	1,387	2,133	3,408
Speech Impaired					
Total	1,995	913	555	315	212
Male	1,306	606	366	208	127
Female	688	307	189	107	86
Paralysis					
Total	1,532	121	353	470	588
Male	803	67	188	270	279
Female	729	55	165	200	309
Orthopedic Handicap-- Upper Extremities					
Total	2,500	105	934	827	634
Male	1,486	69	671	479	268
Female	1,014	36	264	348	366
Orthopedic Handicap-- Lower Extremities					
Total	7,147	1,124	2,491	1,914	1,618
Male	3,643	634	1,466	951	592
Female	3,503	490	1,025	963	1,025
Absence of Major Extremities					
Total	358	13	70	136	138
Male	252	8	53	109	82
Female	106	6	17	27	56

SOURCE: National Center for Health Statistics, unpublished data from the 1977 Health Interview Survey.

Approximately two-thirds of all reported impairments are in the two categories of "deaf and hearing impaired" (more than 16 million) and "blind and visually impaired" (more than 11 million). Over 7 million people report "orthopedic handicaps" of the lower extremities. With the exception of speech impairments (almost 2 million), the prevalence of impairments increases with age. For most impairments, men outnumber women, but after age 65, the ratio is reversed, presumably because of the greater life expectancy of women.

Persons reporting limitation of activity due to chronic conditions made up approximately 13 percent of the non-institutionalized population in the mid-1970s (Table 23). The data show that limitation of activity increases with age, while more men than women and more blacks than whites report activity limitations. A larger proportion of persons below the poverty level report work disability (which may be the cause of their poverty) than do those with incomes above poverty level.

Estimates of the number of persons handicapped because of "mental impairment" are difficult to make. For psychiatric disorders, persons under active treatment at any particular time are only a part of the population that might properly be included in prevalence figures, and attempts to estimate the prevalence of psychiatric disorders in the community are open to question on several grounds.[11] Nevertheless, some estimates of the prevalence of many psychiatric conditions can be made based upon projections from local studies.

A recent literature review by a committee from the American Psychiatric Assocation provides estimates for a number of conditions. The schizophrenic population is put at approximately 1.1 million persons (of whom an estimated 200,000 are hospitalized). An estimated 600,000-800,000 persons (most of whom are in the community) have manic-depressive disease, and an estimated 600,000-1,250,000 non-institutionalized persons have senile psychoses.[12] More than 250,000 nursing home residents are reported to have mental disorders.[13] Estimates of the number of alcoholics or alcohol abusers range from 9 to 13 million, and estimates (and definitions) of drug abusers vary widely; between 1 and 2 million people are estimated to be "drug dependent."[14] The President's Commission on Mental Health estimates the number of persons with neuroses to be between 20 and 30 million persons, with another 15 million having "personality disorders."[15] Many of these figures are imprecise and of uncertain relevance to Section 504, because such persons are (and should be) unlabeled in the community and, thus, not suffer the discrimination that may follow from the attachment of a label. Although others may respond negatively to their behavior, it seems unlikely that Section 504 will be interpreted to mean that people cannot be treated differently because of their behavior, and it is probably inevitable that people who are, for example, unpleasant to the staff in a hospital will receive less attention from the staff. The attribution of such unpleasantness to "mental impairment," thereby making differential treatment of unpleasant persons a violation of Section 504, does not seem to be a useful direction in which to move.

The mentally retarded population is estimated to include approximately 600,000 moderately, severely, and profoundly retarded persons (IQ below 50) and 2-6 million mildly retarded persons (IQ 50-70). Approximately one-third of retarded persons suffer multiple handicaps, including mental illness, epilepsy, cerebral palsy, and other disabilities.[16]

Table 23. SELF-ASSESSMENT OF HEALTH AND LIMITATION OF ACTIVITY, ACCORDING TO SELECTED CHARACTERISTICS: UNITED STATES, 1977

Characteristic	Self-assessment of health as fair or poor	With limitation of activity			
		Total	Limited but not in major activity	Limited in amount or kind of major activity	Unable to carry on major activity
	Percent of Population				
Total [1,2,3,4]	11.9	13.0	3.0	6.5	3.4
Age					
Under 17 years	4.2	3.4	1.5	1.7	0.2
17-44 years	8.5	8.1	2.8	4.1	1.2
45-64 years	22.0	23.1	4.5	12.3	6.2
65 years and over	29.9	43.0	5.7	20.1	17.2
Sex[2]					
Male	11.4	14.1	3.0	5.2	5.8
Female	12.5	12.0	3.0	7.6	1.5
Race[2]					
White	10.9	12.8	3.1	6.4	3.2
Black	20.8	15.9	2.4	7.9	5.6
Family Income[2]					
Less than $5,000	24.2	22.2	3.9	11.3	7.1
$5,000-$9,999	16.1	15.8	3.0	7.8	4.9
$10,000-$14,999	10.9	12.0	2.9	6.2	2.9
$15,000-$24,999	7.5	10.0	2.9	4.8	2.3
$25,000 or more	5.2	8.8	3.1	4.2	1.5
Geographic region[2]					
Northeast	10.8	12.0	2.8	6.1	3.2
North Central	10.5	12.3	2.9	6.5	2.9
South	15.0	14.0	2.8	7.0	4.1
West	10.0	13.5	3.8	6.3	3.5
Location of residence[2]					
Within SMSA	10.9	12.4	3.0	6.2	3.2
Outside SMSA	14.2	14.2	3.1	7.2	3.9

[1]Data are based on household interviews of a sample of the civilian non-institutionalized population.
[2]Age adjusted by the direct method to the 1970 civilian non-institutionalized population, using 4 age intervals.
[3]Includes all other races not shown separately.
[4]Includes unknown family income.

SOURCE: Division of Health Interview Statistics, National Center for Health Statistics: Data are from the Health Interview Survey and are based on household interviews of a sample of the civilian non-institutionalized population.

ISSUES IN ASSESSING HEALTH CARE PROBLEMS OF HANDICAPPED PERSONS

"Health" and the Limits of the Medical Model

The needs of handicapped persons frequently are for services not properly called "medical," but rather are social, psychological, and/or rehabilitative. Thus, the question of adequacy of services for handicapped persons is not only a question of whether they receive the needed amount of medical services but also whether they receive the appropriate type of services. Proper coordination and priorities in services require attention not only to prevent handicapped persons from being underserved (by not receiving needed diagnostic, therapeutic, or rehabilitative services), but also from being overserved (and unnecessarily losing some degree of independence), or misserved (as by sterilization based upon incorrect assumptions about a handicapped woman's ability to carry or care for a baby).

Use of Health Services

Persons who have conditions that limit their activity make more use of physicians and hospitals than do other persons (Table 24), which would be expected from their greater incidence of acute conditions and the fact that almost half of this population is older than 65. However, such data do not necessarily mean that their health care needs are being adequately served, because data on need for services are generally not available for handicapped and disabled persons. An additional problem in interpreting statistics on use of medical services is that, for some disabling conditions, higher rates of use may indicate poor quality of initial care. For example, a spinal cord injury not properly treated at the outset can increase and protract the care required.

Available data on dental care of disabled persons indicate that the most seriously disabled see a dentist much less often that do other people (Table 24). Although such data do not translate directly into unmet need for care, it seems likely that there are shortcomings in the dental care of disabled persons.

Difficulties of Assessing Need

The variety of disabling conditions listed in the Section 504 regulations makes it necessary to recognize the differences among handicapping conditions as they affect access to and needs for health care. The health care needs of persons with spinal cord injuries differ from those of deaf persons, and deterrents to care for one may not be deterrents for the other. Furthermore, persons with similar handicaps can vary in their needs and the obstacles they encounter because of age, sex, resources, occupation, and the like. Diversity

Table 24. AGE-ADJUSTED PERCENTAGES OR RATES OF SELECTED HEALTH CHARACTERISTICS, BY CHRONIC ACTIVITY LIMITATION STATUS: UNITED STATES, 1974

Health characteristic	Total population	With no limitation of activity	With limitation of activity			
			Total	Limited but not in major activity[1]	Limited in amount or kind of major activity[1]	Unable to carry on major activity[1]
Percent of persons with one or more physician visits within a year of interview[2]	75.3	73.1	87.9	86.0	88.2	90.6
Number of physician visits per person per year[2]	4.9	4.1	10.2	7.3	11.3	14.0
Number of physician visits in the office per person per year[2]	3.4	2.9	6.6	4.9	7.4	8.6
Percent of persons with one or more short-stay hospital episodes within a year of interview[2]	10.7	8.7	21.6	14.4	22.0	41.6
Number of discharges from short-stay hospital per 100 persons per year[2]	14.1	10.5	33.3	18.6	31.8	81.3
Average length of stay for discharges from short-stay hospital[3]	8.4	6.5	12.3	8.2	9.5	19.2
Percent of persons with one or more dental visits within a year of interview[2]	49.3	50.3	47.8	56.8	44.7	30.2
Number of dental visits per person per year[2]	1.7	1.7	1.8	2.1	1.8	1.1
Incidence of acute conditions per 100 persons per year[2]	175.7	170.5	216.9	212.2	232.1	183.0
Number of persons injured per 100 persons per year[2]	28.5	27.1	36.6	31.9	43.6	
Days of restricted activity per person per year[2]	17.2	10.2	50.6	26.1	50.5	100.0
Days of bed disability per person per year[2]	6.7	4.2	18.9	8.5	16.7	48.8

[1]Major activity refers to ability to work, keep house, or engage in school or preschool activities.

[2]Age adjusted, by the direct method to the age distribution of the total, civilian, noninstitutionalized population of the United States.

[3]Age adjusted, by the direct method, to the age distribution of the discharges from short-stay hospitals of the total, civilian, non-institutionalized population of the United States.

SOURCE: Vital and Health Statistics, Series 10, Number 112. National Center for Health Statistics.

among handicapped persons, as well as the variety of services that may be needed, and settings in which they may be provided, greatly complicate the implementation of Section 504 as it affects health care.

Three different types of health care can be distinguished to meet the needs of handicapped persons:

(1) General health care, or "mainstream care" Handicapped and non-handicapped persons share certain basic health care needs and expectations. It is reasonable to expect a blind person with an acute ear infection, for example, to have similar medical needs as would a seeing person with the same condition. Questions of equity or discrimination in such instances would rest on whether there are unreasonable interferences with the individual's ability to get appropriate medical care when needed, not in the nature of the care itself. A possible effect of Section 504 may be to increase the availability of mainstream medical care to handicapped people. That would be consistent with the larger social movement to increase the independence of, and decrease the isolation or segregaton of, handicapped persons in the United States.

(2) General health care that, for some types of handicap, may require special training or facilities to provide A difficulty in attempting to provide mainstream care to handicapped persons is that even the general medical needs of some handicapped persons are best met by professionals who have received specialized training and in facilities that have specialized equipment. Thus, for example, the medical management of the general health care of paraplegic patients is best carried out by physicians who are knowledgeable about the threat of kidney infection. A variety of other examples comes from the field of dental care:

- Persons with Down's syndrome require frequent dental visits and maintenance of good oral hygiene because of their propensity for periodontal disease; yet some also have short attention spans and high anxiety levels, which require special attention and sensitivity by the dentist or dental hygienist.
- Some drugs used to control seizure episodes for individuals with epilepsy also induce excessive gum tissue growth, which can become infected. In treating such individuals, however, the dentist must be prepared to deal with seizures, which may occur during treatment.
- Some persons with cerebral palsy exhibit bruxing, or grinding of the teeth and also may have difficulty swallowing, resulting in rapid buildup of plaque caused by their teeth and gums being continuously bathed in saliva. They may also have continual involuntary movements, which require the dentist to devise methods to safely control such movement in order to provide care.[17]

The care of patients with many chronic diseases is best carried out by specialists. A physician who declines to accept a patient with a condition about which he lacks experience or training might be seen as denying that patient access to mainstream care. However, if such actions are motivated by a concern that the patient receives proper care, it is unlikely that objections would be raised, except perhaps in situations where no appropriate referral is made or where treatment is refused by all sources of care. Nevertheless, this illustrates the complexity of the issues raised by Section 504.

Some general care needs of handicapped persons, needs shared by the general population, can best be met in specialized (non-mainstream) situations. To date, little attention has been given to the question of whether and how to increase access to mainstream care settings and, if so, how also to provide specialized care for needs that handicapped persons share with others. Does Section 504 in principle require providers to be prepared to meet specialized needs associated with certain handicapping conditions? Should, for example, dentists participating in Medicaid be required under Section 504 to treat otherwise eligible patients with cerebral palsy? More important to the intent of Section 504, would the needs of such patients be furthered by regulatory requirements that move in such a direction? A negative answer to such a question, however, need not be considered a categorically negative answer to the question of whether providers should be better prepared to meet the general medical needs of handicapped persons.

Compliance requirements that apply to all providers might be desirable to assure that certain general health care needs of persons with relatively common handicaps are met. Yet such requirements should reflect the fact that some needs are best met by providers with specialized knowledge and facilities, particularly when those needs are infrequent in the population. An alternative approach might seek to ensure that the needed specialized services and knowledge are available in each specified geographic region, even though this is not consistent with the mainstreaming goal.

(3) Specialized treatment or management of the handicapping condition Certain needs of handicapped persons stem directly from their condition and are specific to particular kinds of handicaps. Obtaining services for these needs raises problems of the supply and distribution of appropriate, highly specialized services and manpower. Many persons concerned with the interests of handicapped and chronically disabled persons see serious shortcomings in provision of care, ranging from the treatment of the chronically mentally ill, to the initial therapy of the spinal-cord-injured patient, and the rehabilitation of the person who has had a stroke. The adequacy of societal resources for meeting the specialized needs of certain handicapped and disabled populations may only occasionally raise issues that can be addressed under Section 504, which contains no provisions for funding needed services. Yet that adequacy of resources, along with the soundness and breadth of health professionals' approaches to care, may be of fundamental importance to meeting many of the needs of the handicapped.

Because handicapped persons may have particular needs for care, comparisons of the care received by the handicapped and non-handicapped shed little light on whether there are differences in the receipt of needed care. An assessment of the care of handicapped persons, thus, cannot be based on comparison with patterns of care received by other groups. Comparisons with ideals are more appropriate. In considering this problem, the committee agreed on two tentative bases on which to assess the care of handicapped persons. First, is the care they receive equally effective, in relation to existing knowledge, as the care received by other patients? Second, does the care of handicapped persons unnecessarily restrict their autonomy and independence? While neither of these criteria is readily subject to measurement, each calls attention to an important aspect of the care of people with particular needs. The committee has attempted to make use of these concepts in assessing the care of handicapped persons.

DETERRENTS TO HEALTH CARE FOR HANDICAPPED PERSONS

In this section, we examine deterrents to the use of health care services by handicapped individuals. Although the deterrents most often cited in the literature and in comments received by the committee are discussed individually below, each can operate in concert with others to impede or prevent handicapped persons from obtaining care.

Some of these deterrents can be eliminated by enforcement of Section 504 and its regulations, by education of providers, by efforts to inform and educate handicapped persons of their rights under Section 504, and by programs that may assist them in obtaining needed medical care. However, other deterrents, such as those built into specific programs, may require legislative changes. And some problems can be eliminated only through broader social changes that are relatively unaffected by government regulation.

Attitudes/Knowledge of Health Professionals

Negative or inappropriate attitudes of health professionals toward handicapped persons can be subtle and insidious impediments to care and are among the problems cited most often by handicapped persons and others concerned with their rights. The attitudes of health care personnel are often perceived by handicapped individuals as reflecting insensitivity, lack of concern, and a devaluation of patients as persons. Such attitudes can lead to patient dissatisfaction with health services and to failure of a provider to treat a handicapped person appropriately or even to treat at all.[18]

The problem of attitude is complex and is not confined to health professionals. Persons with visible handicaps have long been treated with a mixture of fear, uneasiness, and paternalism and have often been subject to discrimination because of assumptions about their "differences." Biases against the different obviously can and do operate in the health care sector; at the extremes this can be seen in instances of lesser efforts being made to resuscitate alcoholics or resistance to actively treating complications in newborns with Down's syndrome.[19]

Other factors that can influence attitudes of care by providers include ignorance or lack of familiarity with certain handicapping conditions, which may result in lack of confidence and fears of inadequacy in treating such persons[20] and, perhaps, also fears of malpractice; the traditional emphasis in medicine on acute illness and "healing," which leads some physicians to view the chronically disabled as "failures" of medicine and be disinclined to accept them as patients; and the tendency of physicians to address the needs of handicapped persons in narrow medical terms, rather than in terms of broader social support.

Some providers treat handicapped persons in an overprotective fashion that encourages unnecessary dependency, failing to recognize that "disability does not mean inability."[21] While such complaints are not unique to handicapped persons, excessively paternalistic treatment is viewed by many of the handicapped population as potentially destructive of their desire to be as independent as possible.[22] It may also cause providers to fail to recognize that their patients' own knowledge and experience in dealing with their handicap is a valuable source of information that can be used beneficially in their care.[23] An example offered in testimony to the committee was the case of a spinal-cord-injured patient whose knowledge of his body's idiosyncratic responses to infection was ignored by health professionals who incorrectly interpreted those responses as symptoms of an adverse drug reaction.[24] Similarly, persons capable of managing their own catheterization outside of the hospital may not be allowed to do so as inpatients because the staff assumes they are incapable.

In order to promote more appropriate attitudes and care, many commentators have called for better training of health professionals to meet the medical, rehabilitative, and psychosocial needs of handicapped persons.[25] Studies of dentists show, for example, that providers who receive instruction in the care of handicapped persons as part of their undergraduate or graduate training are more likely to treat such patients in their practices.[26]

Although it is unrealistic to expect all health care personnel to be knowledgeable about the specific needs of all handicapped individuals, the training that health care personnel receive could, nevertheless, help in dispelling myths and stereotypes, in recognizing the differences among handicapping conditions as well as the individual nature of functional capabilities, and in encouraging non-paternalistic attitudes toward handicapped persons. Several questions merit consideration: What training--both in attitudes and skills--should all students receive, and what training is most realistically confined to a specialized subset of health professionals? What methods can be used to incorporate needed training into the curricula? A number of dental schools, for example, have instituted programs for care of the disabled, which might serve as models for other health care professional schools.[27] Additionally, postgraduate education programs on care of handicapped persons could be expanded to sensitize and educate those providers already in practice, as well as to reinforce any earlier training.

Supply and Distribution of Resources and Services

The uneven distribution of health care resources and services in the United States--both geographically and by specialty--is a deterrent to the care for many persons who are handicapped, particularly those in rural and inner city areas where manpower and facilities usually are most scarce. Although Section 504 provisions seem not to be the issue, a number of specific problems have been identified in recent years:

- The Special Populations Subpanel of the President's Commission on Mental Health estimated that only 15 mental health programs for deaf persons existed throughout the United States, none of which were in a community mental health center and only a small number of which were fully functional.[28] In addition, only 20 psychiatrists, 16 psychologists, 19 social workers, and 27 psychiatric nurses were working with deaf persons and few of these personnel were deaf themselves or able to communicate in sign language. The commission concluded that 85 percent of deaf persons needing mental health services were not receiving them because the services were not available.
- Less than 1 percent of all practicing physicians (1,742 in 1977) specialize in physical medicine and rehabilitation.[29] One estimate suggests that demand for physiatrists will exceed supply by 100 percent by 1990.[30]
- The number of personnel providing general health care services to handicapped persons is unknown, nor is it known how many within that group have the knowledge of management and treatment of problems of handicapping conditions to enable them to provide the most appropriate general care. Few health care professional schools offer such training.

One proposed solution to the problem of supply and distribution of health services is to establish multi-disciplinary, comprehensive state/regional treatment centers to meet the needs of the handicapped population, with home care and outreach services made available to persons needing care in rural and remote areas.[31] A variety of other approaches may also be helpful, but the problem deserves serious attention.

Physical Deterrents

Physical deterrents to health care for handicapped persons include a lack of public transportation for the disabled and various types of architectural barriers. These largely are high curbs and stairs that are not negotiable, and doors that are too narrow for persons in wheelchairs. Such barriers prevent some persons from entering buildings or treatment areas and preclude their use of some services. Hospital rooms that are not designed to give persons in wheelchairs access to toilets can limit the ability of some handicapped patients to function independently.

The Architectural Barriers Act of 1968 (P.L. 90-480) requires special design features for handicapped persons in all buildings that receive funding through federal grants or loans. These features include certain numbers and design of parking spaces; walkways and curbs that facilitate movement of wheelchairs or crutches; accessible routes and entrances; and reachable, visible, and audible signals and controls--for example, elevator control buttons accessible to wheelchair occupants, raised letters or numerals at corridor doors to identify each floor for those who are visually handicapped, and audible elevator call signals.[32] Compliance with governmental standards and specifications is enforced by the Architectural and Transportation Barriers Compliance Board, which was established by the Rehabilitation Act of 1973.

In addition, regulations for Section 504 specify that each program or activity of a recipient of federal funds "when viewed in its entirety" be readily accessible to handicapped persons (that is, the regulations do not require a recipient to make each of its existing facilities or every part of a facility accessible and usable to handicapped persons). Compliance may be accomplished, for example, by home visits, assigning aids to beneficiaries, or delivering services at alternate sites that are accessible. New construction or alteration of existing facilities must conform to accessibility standards established by the American National Standards Institute, Inc., examples of which were cited above.[33]

Little information is available about how often architectural barriers impede access to health services, the impact of such barriers, or even the number of facilities or programs that are in compliance with the requirements. (The OCR, DHHS, is responsible for reviewing such compliance in health care settings, but has engaged in no compliance activities to date.) However, architectural barriers were not reported as one of the major barriers to obtaining care by disabled persons in the Health Interview Survey.[39] Although most of the physical plants of most hospitals seem likely to be relatively free of barriers to wheelchairs, it is not known how many settings, such as physician or dental offices, are located in buildings that have architectural barriers. The Section 504 regulations allow federal fund recipients that have fewer than 15 employees, and that are unable to comply with the accessibility provisions without significant alteration to existing facilities, to refer handicapped persons to other providers whose services are accessible.

The inability to get to a health care provider or facility was frequently identified as a problem by disabled persons responding to the Health Interview Survey in 1977.[35] Reports of limitations in obtaining care for this reason were four times as common among the disabled as among the fit. Deficiencies in, or lack of, public transportation systems in accommodating the handicapped can be a formidable barrier to their receiving care, although no data are available on the topic.

The Section 504 regulations for health services do not refer specifically to transportation barriers. The Rehabilitation,

Comprehensive Services, and Developmental Disabilities Amendments of 1978 enable DHHS to provide financial assistance to remove transportation barriers as well as architectural and communication barriers if a study has demonstrated the need for such action, and the President has approved the expenditures of funds for this purpose.[36] Medicaid, which provides medical assistance for many disabled persons, requires that states provide or arrange for transportation if necessary to make all covered services available to all eligible individuals on an equitable basis.[37] This requirement is potentially important for many handicapped persons, but the extent to which states are providing such services in their Medicaid programs is unknown. In some rural communities, for example, it has been alleged that transportation assistance is provided to Medicaid eligible persons only if they satisfy a set of unwritten eligibility requirements and if a welfare worker has some time and is willing to transport them.[38]

In response to Section 504, the Department of Transportation issued regulations that pertain to the accessibility of buses and subway cars to wheelchair users. Cost factors have made this requirement controversial, and legislation has been proposed to allow localities to set up alternative transit services for handicapped residents. The issue here is similar to other situations in which mainstream accommodation is at stake: when is it reasonable to serve the needs of handicapped persons through separate or specialized facilities rather than making the adaptations necessary to meet those needs in the general or mainstream system?

Communication Deterrents

Many persons are limited in their ability to communicate, some severely so, because of varying types and degrees of hearing and speech impairments and conditions. Communication problems in health care settings can result in patients' needs being ignored or misunderstood, with possibly serious consequences. For example, communication difficulties associated with handicaps have been alleged to have resulted in erroneous diagnoses of mental retardation.[39] Dissatisfaction with health services and a reluctance to seek care when needed may result not only from difficult communication, but also from patients being treated as intellectually deficient or emotionally disturbed.[40]

Estimates of the number of people with speech difficulties are quite imprecise, ranging from 1 million to 8 million persons (Table 22).[41] The type of aid that persons in this population need to facilitate communication in a health care setting depends upon their specific speech impairment.

Impairment of hearing is the single most prevalent impairment in the United States, although estimates of the number of persons with some type of hearing loss vary widely (Table 22).[42] The National Association of the Deaf estimates that there are 14.5 million people who can be considered hearing impaired (with some degree of hearing loss in one or both ears). Seven million of these have significant bilateral loss (substantial difficulty hearing in both ears) and 2 million can be considered deaf (cannot hear or understand speech). Of these 2 million deaf persons, approximately 450,000 are prevocationally deaf (they become deaf prior to 19 years of age); this population is most likely to communicate through such modes as sign. Forty percent of all hearing impairments occur in the population 65 years or older (Table 22).[43] The diversity of the hearing-impaired population has important implications for the modes of communication that are feasible for particular patients, since proficiency in both English and in sign language is related to age at onset of deafness and to education.

Under traditional assumptions, persons with hearing impairments have been viewed as responsible for assuring that communication can take place, either via written notes or by bringing someone with them to help them communicate. Health providers were thus absolved of responsibility for assuring effective communication with such patients.[44] By contrast, the Section 504 regulations place the responsibility for communication with the provider. Hospitals that are covered by the law and that provide emergency care must ensure that means are available for communicating effectively with persons who have impaired hearing and who require emergency treatment. In addition, recipients of federal funds who employ 15 or more persons are required to provide appropriate auxiliary aids to persons with sensory, manual, or speaking disabilities where necessary to ensure that such persons are not denied appropriate benefits or services because of their handicap. Examples of such aids include braille and tape-recorded material for the blind and interpreting for the deaf. Smaller providers also may be required to provide such aids where it would not adversely affect their ability to provide services.

Although such auxiliary aids are legally required, and the hearing-impaired population is large, no systematic information is available regarding the extent to which hearing- or speech-impaired persons are unable to obtain adequate health care because of communication problems. Some recorded cases represent situations that are not precisely addressed by the regulations, such as deaf persons unsuccessfully seeking treatment at hospital clinics or alcohol treatment centers, but not in emergency situations as addressed by the regulations. In other instances, the regulations have apparently been ignored, as in the case of a deaf woman with a skull fracture who was sent home from an emergency room in Chicago because the hospital refused to provide an interpreter.[45]

Although interpreters are one type of auxiliary aid that could be made available to hearing-impaired persons in health care facilities, the committee could locate no studies that show (1) what proportion of the hearing-impaired population would be able to take advantage of the services of interpreters were they available or (2) what impact interpreters have on health status and satisfaction with care. Some clues as to how hearing-impaired persons presently cope with communication problems in seeking health care come from a recent survey of deaf activists. (No comparable data are available for a more representative sample of deaf persons.) The majority of these persons reported that they relied on written communication with hospital personnel, although the authors noted that writing is "more likely to lead to misunderstanding than sign language interpretation," and the majority of adults deafened in childhood expressed confidence in their ability to sign and to read sign.[46] (This agrees with an earlier, broader survey of prevocationally deaf persons, the majority of whom rated highly their manual communication skills.[47]) Written communication can present serious problems for many deaf persons, particularly for persons deafened in early childhood, since their proficiency in English may be limited. With regard to reading ability, for example, deaf adults average fourth grade level.[48] However, respondents to this survey encountered interpreters in the health care setting only 8 percent or less of the time.[49]

This low figure might be a reflection of the fact that the number of certified interpreters in the country currently is approximately 2,000 persons.[50] A number of other factors further complicate the provision of interpreters for deaf persons. One is the distinction between individuals who use sign language and those who read lips or use other forms of communication not involving sign language.[51] The belief that lip-readers do not need assistance in communicating is often unfounded; many lip-readers understand less than half of what is being said. The potential for misunderstandings is therefore substantial. Furthermore, many interpreters are not trained in both signing and oral interpreting, so communication problems may remain even in health care settings in which an interpreter is present. A less common problem concerns ethnic individuals who are hearing impaired and who use other than American Sign Language (sign languages differ as do spoken languages).[52] A final problem in the use of interpreters is the question of privacy and confidentiality in the doctor/patient relationship. The National Registry of Interpreters for the Deaf, a national certifying organization for interpreters, does have a code of ethics that requires that interpreters protect any confidence to which they are privy.

Financing Health Care

The cost of health services was identified by disabled persons in the 1977 Health Interview Survey as a major obstacle to obtaining care.[53] Government health care programs and private health insurance do not remove this obstacle for many handicapped persons.

An array of health service programs exists for handicapped persons at federal, state, and local levels, including rehabilitation programs, community health and mental health centers, and programs for narrowly specified beneficiaries. There are important programs for the handicapped in the Department of Defense and the Veterans Administration, but most programs at the federal level come under the DHHS. Medicare, Medicaid, and Crippled Children's Services are three major health care programs serving handicapped persons. Examination of the deterrents to care that are built into these programs raises that are built into these programs raises the question of whether federal and state governments, in the face of finite resources and competing interests, are in a broad sense discriminating against substantial segments of the handicapped population.

Medicare is the federal health insurance program for the aged, certain disabled persons, and those suffering from chronic renal failure. The eligibility requirements and benefit structure are the same throughout the country and apply without regard to income or assets. It is administered as an insurance program. Part A of Medicare is available to persons when they reach age 65 and to those with chronic renal disease requiring dialysis or renal transplant regardless of age. Part A covers hospital services, skilled nursing home care, and home health visits for a specified number of days or number of visits.

All persons aged 65 and over and all persons enrolled in Part A may elect to enroll in Part B of Medicare, which pays for physician visits, laboratory and X-ray services, outpatient hospital care, and additional home health care visits. Part B is financed by a modest monthly premium charge on enrollees and by federal taxes. It has been suggested, however, that the deductible and coinsurance features of Part B act as a deterrent to obtaining services under Medicare by the poor, who include disproportionate numbers of disabled persons.[54] Furthermore, although Part B services are those most likely to meet the general health care needs of handicapped persons, providers under the program are not deemed by DHHS to be receiving federal financial assistance and are exempt from the Section 504 regulations.[55]

Disabled persons become eligible for Medicare benefits after they have been entitled to Social Security Disability Insurance (SSDI) benefits (based on a period of covered employment) for two years. Eligibilty for the latter benefits is contingent on a determination that the individual is "incapable of engaging in any substantial gainful activity because of a medically determinable physical or mental impairment that has lasted or can be expected to last continuously for at least 12 months or to result in death."[56] When the initial 5-month period for determining disability under the disability insurance program is included, a waiting period of 29 months exists between the onset of a disabling condition and eligibility for benefits under Medicare, although in some instance coverage may be obtained under Medicaid.

The waiting period was enacted in an effort to limit program costs and to direct Medicare coverage to those whose disabilities have proved to be severe and long lasting.[57] However, this means that Medicare benefits are not available during the initial, often acute, phase of disability when health services are particularly needed. For example, SSDI beneficiaries in 1974 not eligible for Medicare used almost twice as many hospital days and physician visits as eligible beneficiaries.[58] Early treatment may greatly affect the eventual severity of some disabilities. As an example, early placement of persons with spinal cord injuries into a medical rehabilitation program has been shown to reduce the severity of the disability.[59]

Until quite recently, disabled persons eligible for Medicare who returned to work and then suffered a relapse had to re-establish their Medicare eligibility in an additional 24-month waiting period. This provision, which was quite inconsistent with the goal of maximizing the independence of disabled persons, was altered by the Social Security Disability Amendments of 1980, which did away with the waiting period and extended Medicare coverage for four years after a disabled person returns to work instead of one year.[60]

Other problems and gaps in coverage under Medicare are likely to have a disproportionate effect on handicapped persons and bring into focus the conflict that can arise between cost considerations and the goals of Section 504:

- No coverage for optical aids, hearing aids, or dental care;[61] limitations on hospital services (up to 90 days), which may constitute inadequate lengths of stay for those with severe disabilities, such as quadriplegia, paraplegia, and multiple amputations. Spinal-cord-injured people may need 120 days for the first stay.
- Limitations on skilled nursing home care (100 days per benefit period, preceded by at least 3 days of hospitalization), which makes many disabled persons, particularly the elderly disabled, convert to Medicaid, with its attendant disincentives to providers and resulting discrimination (see Chapter 3).
- Limitations on home health care visits (100 visits), which may force a person into an institution.
- Limited psychiatric benefits, such as coverage restricted to a lifetime maximum of 190 days of inpatient psychiatric hospitalization, and a limit on annual payments for ambulatory services of $250 per patient.[62]

Medicaid is a federal-state matching grant program providing medical assistance for low-income persons who also meet certain eligibility requirements (for example, aged, blind, disabled, or members of families with dependent children). All states except Arizona currently participate in the program. Each state administers and operates its own program, and, subject to federal guidelines, determines eligibility and scope of benefits. States participating in Medicaid are required to offer inpatient and outpatient hospital services; laboratory and X-ray services; skilled nursing home care; home health care; physician services; family planning services; and early and periodic screening, diagnosis, and treatment (EPSDT) for children under age 21, as well as to arrange for or provide transportation to needed services. States may also provide a wide variety of optional services (for example, drugs and dental care), but the amount and extent of such services vary widely from state to state.

Eligibility requirements also vary from state to state. Thus, disabled persons eligible for services in one state can be ineligible in another. Eligibility is often linked to actual or potential receipt of cash assistance under federally assisted welfare programs, but states do have the option of covering the medically needy--those with incomes adequate to purchase food, clothing, and housing, but not adequate to meet the cost of medical care. Anyone receiving Supplemental Security Income (SSI) is eligible; the definition of disability under SSI is the same as that for disability insurance, except that disability for children is evaluated in terms of such factors as growth, maturation of physical and functional characteristics, and emotional and social development.[63]

For disabled persons who qualify, the program creates unfortunate disincentives for employment. Although employment is important to the independence of handicapped individuals, earnings above certain, often low levels result in the loss of eligibility for Medicaid services on which they may be dependent for meeting substantial medical expenses. Such persons must either find a lower-paying job in order to retain benefits, quit work, or attempt to cover their medical expenses as best they can. This is made more difficult by the fact that the health insurance connected with employment often inadequately covers expenses associated with chronic problems and excludes costs associated with treatment of conditions that existed prior to coverage. Thus, the person who has been disabled by a chronic condition may find that the costs associated with the loss of Medicaid are so prohibitive as to make returning to work not feasible.

A number of other features of the Medicaid program can result in eligible, disabled people having difficulty in getting needed care. As was described in Chapter 2, many providers are unwilling to accept Medicaid recipients as patients, citing as reasons inadequate reimbursement levels and delays in payment. In addition, fixed reimbursement levels for units of care, such as an office visit or a day of care, create disincentives to care for persons whose needs in terms of time, facilities, or personnel are greater than average. Many handicapped and disabled persons fall into that category. The President's Commission on Mental Health noted that reimbursement rates for community mental health centers and/or psychiatrists are so low that many providers refuse to participate in Medicaid and needed mental health services are not available to poor people who are mentally handicapped.[64]

Although all states are required to provide EPSDT services for all Medicaid recipients under 21, a study of that program by the Children's Defense Fund found that the program is especially inadequate for eligible handicapped children. Such children often become eligible for Medicaid, at least in theory, on the basis of their eligibility for the federally administered Supplemental Security Income Program. However, this does not necessarily bring them to the attention of the state-administered Medicaid program, and they may never be told about the EPSDT program. Furthermore, even if they are screened under EPSDT, many of the medical services they may need (such as physical therapy) may not be covered by their state's Medicaid program.[65]

There are also important limitations and variations in benefits from state to state that may affect the services that are available to handicapped persons. All states, for example, provide dental benefits for Medicaid eligible children, but not all provide such benefits for eligible adults.[66] The provision of many services under Medicaid are at the option of the state (such as optical aids and hearing aids) and even if such aids are provided, the state may limit the type and extent of such aids. A visually impaired person may be able to obtain regular eyeglasses, for example, but those with special problems may get limited services--the person with albumism may need a change of lenses several times per year but may only be covered for the initial lenses. Or the state may provide a hearing impaired person with only one hearing aid when two are needed.

In some instances, states are accused of using subjective criteria to distinguish between the "deserving" and the "nondeserving," and factors such as age or severity of disability may be used in determining whether certain aids will be provided to disabled persons. One commentator alleges that in California electric wheelchairs appear to be made available only to persons in their 20s.[67] Little attention has as yet been given to the question of whether the rationing of scarce resources on the basis of need (or on predictions regarding likelihood to benefit) is inconsistent with Section 504.

Mental health services under Medicaid, as under Medicare, are limited. For example, limitations on payments, age, and services exclude persons between the ages of 21 and 65 from Medicaid reimbursement for treatment in a psychiatric facility, because such care has traditionally been a state responsibility. Furthermore, facilities in which more than half of the residents are mentally ill are subject to the "50 percent rule," which classifies them as psychiatric institutions and therefore subject to special restrictions and limitations on reimbursement. With regard to children, maintenance and services are both reimbursed for those in institutions, but only medical care is covered for those in less-restrictive settings. Coupled with the lack of mandated coverage for home health care services for those under 21 (such services are mandatory for adults), a disincentive for deinstitutionalizaton of mentally handicapped children is created.[68]

<u>Crippled Children's Services</u> Title V of the Social Security Act authorizes a program of formula grants to state health agencies for Crippled Children's Services to extend and improve services to handicapped children and to those suffering from conditions that lead to crippling, particularly in rural and economically depressed areas. Notwithstanding its title, the program now covers almost all types of medical problems. Services provided include locating handicapped children and providing medical, surgical, corrective and other assistance for diagnosis, hospitalization, and post-hospitalization care.

The federal statute does not specify either the amount or type of service that states may provide under this program or what conditions are considered "crippling." A crippled child is defined as "an individual under the age of 21 who has an organic disease, defect, or condition which may hinder the achievement of normal growth and development" (P.L. 94-271). All children so defined are eligible for diagnostic services. Treatment services are provided to children in financially needy families, with determination of financial need left to each state.[69] Benefits under the programs, however, cease at age 21, despite the fact that most such conditions are permanent. Coverage of medical expenses thereafter depends on the individual's or the family's resources or eligibility for other public programs.

States report annually on conditions treated in children served by the program, and this information provides a minimal definition of what conditions may be covered or excluded in the reporting state. Figures for 1973 federal expenditures per client on a state-by-state basis ranged from a low of $26.90 in Washington, D.C., to a high of $249.17 in Ohio.[70] Large state-by-state variations also exist in the types of conditions covered within the program.[71] In 1976, for example, Iowa reported that 22.9 percent of its caseload was mental, psychoneurotic, and personality disorders, but California reported none. Indiana led all other states with 49.8 percent of its total caseload reported as multiply handicapped, compared with a national average for the program of 24.2 percent, and North Dakota reported the lowest proportion--2.5 percent--as similarly handicapped.[72] It is not clear in materials reviewed by the committee whether such variations are artifacts of variations in data-reporting systems or are due to state-level decisions to exclude certain types of handicapped children from this program and, if so, whether such exclusions stem from coverage of these types of children in other programs is not apparent.

Although these three programs--Medicare, Medicaid, and Crippled Children's Services--are all intended to meet the health care needs of the disabled population, each meets only certain needs and has its own constituency and interests. Thus, each not only fails to serve "a significant portion of its potential clientele,"[73] but may be poorly serving many of its beneficiaries as well.

<u>Private health insurance</u> also is of obvious importance in the financing of health care. Policies often exclude coverage for "pre-existing conditions"--medical conditions present when a policy is taken out. This exclusion also can apply to children born with such conditions, even though the parents have health insurance coverage for themselves.[74] Some insurance companies cover persons who have such conditons by underwriting "substandard risks"--those who for several reasons do not qualify for standard coverage. One way to underwrite such risks is a waiver or rider exempting coverage for a specific disability or form of physical impairment affecting a specified part of the body. A problem in such coverage arises when a person is hospitalized or disabled for another condition that might be construed by the insurer to be directly or indirectly caused by the waivered disability. Additional methods for underwriting substandard risks include extending the elimination period (the period for which the insurer is not responsible) and offering coverage with extra premium payments.[75] It is not clear to what extent practices that result in no coverage or higher premiums for handicapped or disabled people have a sound actuarial basis rather than being based on guesses and assumptions.

Health insurance coverage may be available to handicapped persons who are employed through group coverage at the workplace. However, the job mobility of persons with chronic conditions (particularly those whose chronic condition developed while they were employed) may be severely constrained by questions about whether they (or their chronic condition) would be covered by insurance in a new place of work. This problem may also apply to employees who have handicapped dependents. An additional problem with handicapped dependents is that parents' insurance coverage for a handicapped child may expire when the child reaches 18 or 21.

The problem of inadequate or unavailable insurance coverage also may lead a handicapped person not to seek employment at all, because of the possibility that their earnings will make them ineligible for public assistance programs, but be inadequate to cover their medical expenses. The cost of care for cystic fibrosis, as just one example, often exceeds $10,000 per person per year and may even exceed $100,000.[76]

Although estimates exist of the number of persons in the United States with or without some form of private health insurance coverage, no current estimates are available to determine how many handicapped persons are in each of these groups. Furthermore, the committee could locate no information regarding such matters as how many handicapped persons are covered for most or all medical costs associated with the handicapping condition, how many are paying extra premiums to cover handicap-related care, or how many have coverage that excludes such care. The major studies of how people finance their medical expenses, including the recent National Health Expenditure Survey conducted by the National Center for Health Services Research, have not collected data that would allow separate analysis of the experiences and practices of handicapped and disabled persons. Although some difficult sampling problems would have to be overcome for a national survey of this population, questions about the health status of the handicapped population, whether and where they obtain care, and how they pay for it seem too important to be ignored in the future.

Medical screens Handicapped persons who may be unable to acquire private health insurance because of pre-existing conditions may face similar medical screens in certain government-assisted programs, namely, prepaid community health centers and federally qualified health maintenance organizations (HMOs). Prospective individual members may be reviewed with regard to their probable future need for continued, long-term treatment of an illness or condition--a distinct probability for many handicapped persons--and if their potential need and use of services are high, they may be excluded from participation in these programs. Medical screens resulting in handicapped persons being denied membership specifically because of their handicapping condition, however, would appear to be inconsistent with Section 504.

The rationale for medical screens is one of economics. Such practices limit the organization's financial risk (potential health service costs) by using actuarial predictions of costs and establishing of capitation rates sufficient to meet those costs, enabling the organization to compete effectively in the health care market. Some health centers have contended that medical screens are necessary for their economic survival. The OCR has argued that a center's use of a medical screen is discriminatory under both Section 504 and Section 330(a) of Title III of the Public Health Service Act, which requires centers to serve all persons in their catchment areas, regardless of medical condition,[77] but the issue is still unresolved.

In contrast, HMOs, which are subject to Title XIII of the Public Health Service Act, are not required to serve all persons in their catchment areas, although they must serve all group members, regardless of health status. HMOs, however, medically screen individuals on grounds of protecting their financial viability. Only during an open enrollment period must an HMO accept all individuals who apply (with the exception of those confined to an institution) without regard to health status.*

The OCR is investigating whether medical screens are essential to the economic survival of HMOs and, if so, what the limitations should be on these screens to ensure that such organizations do not discriminate against those who are handicapped. The question remains open on how to reconcile the requirements of Section 504 with the shaky financial status and competitive position of many HMOs. If, in pursuing its goal of encouraging and supporting the development of HMOs, the government exempts HMO medical screens from Section 504, this would raise questions about the government's responsibility for the social goal of non-discrimination and would preempt a more deliberative attempt to reconcile certain economic realities of government programs with the mandate of civil rights.

Long-term care Nursing homes are one of several types of facilities available to meet the long-term care needs of physically and mentally handicapped individuals, particularly the disabled elderly. Questions can be raised, however, about a number of apparently discriminatory practices and policies at both the nursing home and governmental levels.

Witnesses appearing at meetings of the committee reported that handicapped individuals in nursing homes often receive fewer services and lower quality of care than other residents and in some instances are even denied basic services. One report stated that 70 percent of

---

*However, not all HMOs are required to have open enrollment periods. Only those organizations that either have provided comprehensive health services on a prepaid basis for at least five years or have an enrollment of at least 50,000 members, and which did not have a financial deficit in the preceding fiscal year, are required to have an open enrollment period. Furthermore, there are limitations on the duration of the open enrollment period, and the open enrollment requirements may be waived if an HMO demonstrates that compliance would jeopardize its existence.[78]

the patients in skilled nursing facilities needing physical therapy and 90 percent of those needing occupational and speech therapy did not receive them.[79]

The handicapped or disabled person seeking nursing home care may be refused admission because of their needs for care. It is widely recognized that persons who require, or who are assumed will require, "heavy care" are screened out by nursing homes. Such individuals could include blind or deaf persons, those with colostomies, ileostomies, or catheters, as well as those with drug or alcohol problems--in other words, various types of patients who fall within the Section 504 definition of handicapped. Only scattered documentation is available, however, regarding the extent to which this occurs.

The possibility of exclusion of such individuals increases if they are Medicaid recipients. Most nursing homes have long waiting lists and can decide which public and private patients to admit, as well as what rates to charge the private patients. As was described in Chapter 3, state Medicaid payments to nursing homes are often much lower than rates paid by private patients. Because of this disparity, as a recent General Accounting Office report notes, "nursing homes generally prefer to accept private pay applicants over Medicaid applicants and the less disabled over the highly impaired, difficult to care for patient."[80] The New York State Moreland Act Commission investigation into nursing homes observed that many facilities "make it a policy to accept only relatively well patients.[81] Several homes employ 'headhunters' whose task it is not only to find patients to fill beds, but also, and importantly, to screen out difficult cases." It is thus difficult for Medicaid-supported and highly impaired applicants (which in many instances may be identical populations) to find a vacant nursing home bed. This situation is exacerbated in areas where there is a bed shortage.

The use of "heavy-care" criterion by nursing homes to screen out the disabled has yet to be thoroughly examined, but a number of issues bear scrutiny. The heavy-care criterion is apparently applied on an informal basis by nursing homes and is nowhere fully defined.[82] Heavy-care could refer to needs for extensive medical care or personal assistance, or both. It could refer to patients whose personalities or behavior make them more difficult to cope with by staff or other residents. Do all patients classified as heavy-care actually require such care? Are certain conditions routinely assumed to require more care, despite the fact that conditions and functional levels differ among patients?

The economic rationale for screening these patients raises other questions. Are such patients merely less profitable than others, or will the facility actually lose money because the reimbursement rate is inadequate to support the necessary care for these persons? Whether the source of discrimination is seen to lie in federal/state reimbursement policies or in the practices of facilities, a fairer distribution among nursing homes of heavy-care patients and/or Medicaid recipients appears necessary to ensure that handicapped persons needing nursing home care are more readily admitted. If they are in hospitals waiting to be admitted to nursing homes, they may be there for long periods of time, receiving more care than necessary and at considerable public expense;[83] if they are at home, without sufficient care, their condition may be adversely affected.[84]

In contrast to the situation in which handicapped persons are denied admission to nursing homes, many others, particularly the marginally disabled, are being inappropriately placed in such institutions. The nursing home often is used as a housing alternative because of insufficient economic or social resources in the community.[85] The lack of proper facilities is reinforced by the bias toward institutionalization under Medicaid. Although skilled nursing facility care and home health services are mandatory under Medicaid, the states can limit the amount and types of services provided, as well as the reimbursement rates. Most have restricted home health services.[86] On the other hand, despite complaints regarding low reimbursement rates under Medicaid, nursing home participation in Medicaid is quite extensive. The result may not only be more costly in financial terms for society as a whole, but deleterious for the patient. Too often, marginally disabled persons are relegated to nursing homes where little effort is made to meet their personal, social, or rehabilitative needs, thereby reducing their ability and desire to function at their full potential.

CONCLUSIONS

The committee's review of the health care of handicapped persons leaves little doubt that a variety of problems exist, although it is difficult to know the extent to which discrimination in a strict sense is involved. A full statement of the extent and sources of these problems is prevented by the lack of a clear operational definition (or set of definitions) of a "handicapped person" for the purpose of the law and by lack of adequate information about the health status and health care of handicapped persons, whatever definitions may be used.

The committee concluded that present informational inadequacies are partially rooted in priorities and apathy about the condition of handicapped people and partially in conceptual and methodological difficulties. The former problem is symbolized by the failure to collect any information about handicaps in the 1980 census, a matter that should be corrected in 1990, and by the lack of a clear locus of responsibility for assuring that opportunities are taken to collect relevant information. The OCR, because of its responsibilities under Section 504, may be able to play a useful role as a catalyst for bringing about needed improvements in information by working with statistical agencies within the Department of Health and Human Services to increase attention to the topic.

Conceptually, the most fundamental problem is the lack of clear and consistent definitions for use in compiling information about handicapped beneficiaries in federal programs and in collecting information by surveys. Ideally, such a definition should be as consistent as is feasible with the central elements of the Section 504 definition of a handicap: an impairment that significantly limits a person in a major life activity (not just in terms of work disability). (It should also be made clear that temporary impairments or acute conditions are not included.) The need to develop a clear and consistent definition for statistical purposes should be given serious attention, perhaps through the National Committee on Vital and Health Statistics that advises the Secretary of DHHS.

At the same time, more explicit attention should be given to collecting information about the problems experienced by handicapped persons in obtaining health care under available definitions. Consideration should be given to developing standard questions about handicaps that can be included in any general health survey of sufficient size and be used in the presentation of results. In addition, more specific information is needed about the sources of care of handicapped persons and the problems they face in obtaining care. To be most useful, survey instruments should reflect both the types of handicap-specific problems (such as interpreters for deaf patients) that arise in the Section 504 context and problems (such as distance from specialized facilities or lack of coverage under health insurance) that do not. Information about sources of payment for care and participation in governmental programs will also increase the usefulness of such data-collection efforts. Finally, more information is needed about systematic factors that influence the care that handicapped persons receive. This includes state variations in federally funded programs on which many handicapped persons are dependent and information about planning agencies' activities pertaining to the health care problems of handicapped persons.

The committee has noted that the Section 504 definition itself causes problems for both data collection and enforcement both because of its breadth and vagueness and because of its inclusion of disabilities, chronic (and perhaps acute) diseases, mental disorders, and drug and alcohol abusers. It is unlikely that the health care problems of the chronically ill, for example, will be in any way mitigated by being redefined as problems of handicapped persons. The Section 504 definition leads to a confusion of various issues and makes both research and meaningful enforcement activities (including the definition of discrimination) unnecessarily difficult. The legislative definition bears reconsideration.

As far as the OCR is concerned, the committee suggests that it (1) review definitions of handicapping conditions under existing federal programs, (2) develop a set of functional definitions of handicapping conditions under the existing language of Section 504, and (3) develop, with other relevant bureaus and agencies within DHHS, common definitions for data collection, to be included in on-going statistical surveys.

REFERENCES

1. The Rehabilitation Act of 1973, §504, 29 U.S.C. §794 (1976).

2. The Rehabilitation Act Amendments of 1974, §III, 29 U.S.C. 706(6)(1976).
3. 42 Federal Register 22685 (May 4, 1977).
4. Frank Bowe, Handicapping America: Barriers to Disabled People (New York: Harper and Row, 1978) p. 155.
5. 42 Federal Register 22678 (May 4, 1977).
6. Bowe; Lawrence Haber, Identifying the Disabled: Concepts and Methods in the Measurement of Disability, Report No. 1, Social Security Survey of the Disabled, 1966 (Washington, D.C.: DHEW, 1967); Saad Z. Nagi, Disability and Rehabilitation (Columbus, OH: Ohio State University Press, 1969); The Urban Institute, Report of the Comprehensive Service Needs Study (Washington, D.C.: The Urban Institute, 1975).
7. U.S. Department of Health, Education, and Welfare, "Proposals to Reduce the Inconsistencies in Concepts, Criteria, and Definitions of Disability and Handicap," decision memorandum to the Secretary from the Assistant Secretary for Planning and Evaluation (April 7, 1978).
8. The Urban Institute, p. 32; Monroe Berkowitz, "Public Policy Towards Disability--the Numbers, the Programs and Some Economic Problems," in Science and Technology in the Service of the Physically Handicapped, Volume II, Supporting Papers, National Academy of Sciences (Washington, D.C. National Research Council, 1976) p. 37.
9. Rehab Group, Inc., Digest of Data on Persons with Handicaps and Disabilities (Falls Church, VA: Rehab Group, Inc., 1979) p. 1.
10. Social Security Administration, Work Disability in the United States: A Chartbook (Washington, D.C.: Government Printing Office, 1977).
11. President's Commission on Mental Health, "The Burden of Mental Disorders," in Task Panel Reports, Volume II, Appendix (Washington, D.C.: Government Printing Office, 1978) pp. 13-17.
12. The Ad Hoc Committee on the Chronic Mental Patient, "Problems, Solutions, and Recommendations for a Public Policy," in John A. Talbott (ed.), The Chronic Mental Patient (Washington, D.C.: American Psychiatric Association, 1978) pp. 13-15.
13. National Center for Health Statistics, The National Nursing Home Service: 1977 Summary for the United States, Vital and Health Statistics, Series 13, No. 43 (Washington, D.C.: Government Printing Office, 1979) p. 31.
14. The Ad Hoc Committee on the Chronic Mental Patients, p. 14; Thomas R. Vischi et al., The Alcohol, Drug Abuse, and Mental Health National Data Book, DHEW Publication No. (AOM)80-938, (Washington, D.C.: Government Printing Office, 1980) pp. 15-19.
15. The President's Commission on Mental Health, p. 16.
16. President's Committee on Mental Retardation, "A Renewed National Commitment" in Task Panel Reports, Report of the Liaison Task Panel on Mental Retardation, Volume IV, Appendix (Washington, D.C.: Government Printing Office, 1978) p. 2022.
17. Robert Wood Johnson Foundation, Special Report: Dental Care for Handicapped Americans (Princeton, NJ: Robert Wood Johnson Foundation, 1979) pp. 4 and 6.

18. James H. Murphy, Jr. (United Cerebral Palsy Association, Washington, D.C.), personal communication, February 5, 1980; 42 Federal Register 22,686 (May 4, 1977).
19. David Sudnow, Passing On: The Social Organization of Dying (Englewood Cliffs, NJ: Prentice-Hall, 1967) pp. 100-105; Glenn Affleck, "Physicians' Attitudes Toward Discretionary Medical Treatment of Down's Syndrome Infants," Mental Retardation 18 (April 1980) pp. 79-81.
20. Herbert Cohen, "Obstacles to Developing Community Services for the Mentally Retarded" in M. J. Begab and S. A. Richardson (eds.), The Mentally Retarded and Society: A Social Science Perspective, (Baltimore, MD: University Press, 1975) p. 410.
21. Donald Elisburg and Bonnie Friedman, "A Minority Whose Time Has Come," Human Rights 9 (Spring 1980) p. 30-33, 53-54.
22. Hal Kirshbaum (Center for Independent Living, Berkeley, California), personal communication, January 22, 1980; Gregg Downey, "The Disabled Fight for Their Own Cause," Modern Health Care (February 1975) pp. 22 and 24; Joan Rogers and Joanne Ligone, "Psycho-social Parameters in Treating the Person with Quadriplegia," American Journal of Occupational Therapy 33 (July 1979) p. 436.
23. Mark Ozer (Mainstream, Inc., Washington, D.C.), personal communication, April 4, 1980; Downey, pp. 22-23.
24. Ozer.
25. White House Conference on Handicapped Individuals, Final Report, Volume Two: Part A (Washington, D.C.: Government Printing Office, 1977) pp. 29-30; President's Committee on Employment of the Handicapped, National Health Care Policies for the Handicapped (Washington, D.C.: The White House, 1978) p. 41; Downey, p. 23; Albert Pimentel, (National Association of the Deaf, Silver Spring, Maryland), personal communication, January 9, 1980; Irene Leigh, "The Impact of a Hearing Loss on Health Care of the Infant or Preschool Child," Volta Review 77 (January 1975) p. 51.
26. Doris Stiefel, "Inclusion of a Program of Instruction in the Care of the Disabled in a Dental School Curriculum" Journal of Dental Education 43 (1979) p. 262; and Robert E. Roberts et al., "Dental Care for Handicapped Children Reexamined: I. Dental Training and Treatment of the Handicapped," Journal of Public Health Dentistry 38 (Winter 1978) p. 25.
27. Robert Wood Johnson Foundation; Stiefel; Steven Randell and Lawrence Cohen, "Dental Service Established With Minimum Effort" Hospitals 54 (January 1980) pp. 105-107.
28. President's Commission on Mental Health, "Report of the Special Populations Subpanel Mental Health of Physically Handicapped Americans," in Volume III, Appendix (Washington, D.C.: Government Printing Office, 1978) pp. 1003-1004.
29. U.S. Department of Health, Education, and Welfare, Health United States 1979, DHEW Publication No. (PHS) 80-1232 (Washington, D.C.: Government Printing Office, 1980) p. 259.
30. President's Committee on Employment of the Handicapped, p. ix.
31. White House Conference on Handicapped Individuals, p. 30.

32. U.S. Department of Health, Education, and Welfare, Minimum Requirements of Construction and Equipment for Hospitals and Medical Facilities, DHEW Publication No. (HRA) 79-14500 (Washington, D.C.: Government Printing Office, 1979) pp. 1-2.
33. 42 Federal Register 22,681 (May 4, 1977).
34. Jacob J. Feldman (National Center for Health Statistics), Unpublished data from 1977 Health Interview Survey presented to IOM Committee, February 8, 1980.
35. Ibid.
36. U.S. Department of Health, Education, and Welfare, A Summary of Selected Legislation Relating to the Handicapped 1977-78, DHEW Publication No. (OHDS) 79-22003 (Washington, D.C.: Government Printing Office, May 1979) p. 6.
37. Commerce Clearing House, Medicare and Medicaid Guide (Chicago, IL, 1977).
38. Sara Rosenbaum (Children's Defense Fund, Washington, D.C.), Testimony before IOM Committee, Washington, D.C., June 6, 1980.
39. Janet Brown and Martha Redden, A Research Agenda on Science and Technology for the Handicapped (Washington, D.C.: American Association for the Advancement of Science, 1979) p. 28.
40. Russell Love, "Breaking the Sound Barrier" Human Rights 9 (Spring 1980) p. 28.
41. Brown and Redden, pp. 28-29.
42. Michael Marge, "U.S. Service Delivery System for the Hearing Impaired," in L. J. Bradford and W. Hardy (eds.), Hearing and Hearing Impairment (New York: Grune and Stratton, 1979) p. 576.
43. Hal Schwartz (National Association of the Deaf, Silver Spring, Maryland), personal communication, February 21, 1980.
44. Charles D. Goldman, "Open Door Policy" Human Rights 9 (Spring 1980) p. 14.
45. L. Goldberg, "The Law: From Shield to Sword for Deaf People" Human Rights 9 (Spring 1980) p. 51.
46. Jerome Schein and Marcus Delk, "Survey of Health Care for Deaf People" Deaf America (January 1980) pp. 5-6, 27.
47. Jerome Shein and Marcus Delk, The Deaf Population of the United States, (Silver Springs, MD: National Association for the Deaf, 1974).
48. Shein and Delk, 1980, p. 6.
49. Ibid.
50. National Registry of Interpreters for the Deaf (Silver Spring, Maryland), personal communication, May 16, 1980.
51. Brown and Redden, p. 4.
52. Harry Markowicz, American Sign Language: Fact and Fancy, (Washington, D.C.: Gallaudet College, 1977) p. 7.
53. Feldman.
54. Beverlee A. Myers, "Paying for Health Care: The Unequal Burden," Civil Rights Digest 10 (Fall 1977) p. 14.
55 42 Federal Register 22685 (May 4, 1977).
56. 42 U.S.C. §223(d) (1976).
57. United States Code Congressional and Administrative News: House Report No. 92-231, December 26, 1972.

58. President's Committee on Employment of the Handicapped, p. 4.
59. Ibid., p. 7.
60. Social Security Disability Amendments of 1980, Public Law No. 96-265, §103-104, 94 Stat. 441 (1980).
61. U.S. Department of Health, Education, and Welfare, Medicare Handbook, DHEW Publication No. (SSA)-79-10050 (Washington, D.C.: DHEW, 1979) p. 42.
62. President's Commission on Mental Health, Report to the President, Volume I (Washington, D.C.: Government Printing Office, 1978) p. 31.
63. 42 C.F.R. 435 (1979 edition); and Satyon Kachar, "Blind and Disabled Persons Awarded Federally Administered SSI Payments," Social Security Bulletin 42 (June 1979) p. 13.
64. President's Commission on Mental Health, p. 32.
65. Rosenbaum, 1980.
66. Health United States, 1979, p. 128.
67. Marilyn Holle (Western Center for Law and the Handicapped, Los Angeles) Testimony before IOM Committee (Los Angeles, CA, May 9, 1980).
68. President's Commission on Mental Health, "Report of the Task Panel on Legal and Ethical Issues" in Task Panel Reports Volume III, Appendix (Washington, D.C.: Government Printing Office, 1978) pp. 1406-1409.
69. Garry D. Brewer and James Kakalik, Handicapped Children: Strategies for Improving Services (New York: McGraw-Hill, 1979) p. 258.
70. Ibid., p. 258.
71. Ibid., p. 271.
72. U.S. Department of Health, Education, and Welfare, "Crippled Children's Services" (mimeographed data, 1976).
73. Urban Institute, p. 651.
74. B. Greer et al., "Quasi-legal Barriers to Adjustment to Disability: Accident and Hospitaliztion Insurance," Rehabilitation Literature 36 (August 1975) p. 250.
75. Ibid., pp. 274-248.
76. Cystic Fibrosis Foundation, Cystic Fibrosis: A Plea for the Future Volume II (Atlanta, GA: Cystic Fibrosis Foundation, 1978) p. 6.
77. Hal Freeman, Office for Civil Rights, DHHS, personal communication, June 2, 1980.
78. 742 USC, §1301, (d).
79. U.S. Department of Health, Education, and Welfare, Office of Long Term Care, Long Term Care Facility Improvement Study: Introductory Report DHEW Publication No. (O5)76-50021, July 1975.
80. U.S. General Accounting Office, Entering a Nursing Home - Costly Implications for Medicaid and the Elderly (Washington, D.C.: Government Printing Office, 1979) p. 103.
81. New York State Moreland Act Commission on Nursing Homes and Residential Facilities, Long Term Care Regulation: Past Lapses, Future Prospects: A Summary Report. (New York: author, 1976) p. 27.

82. Gretchen Schafft (Foundation of the American College of Nursing Home Administrators, Inc., Bethesda, MD), Testimony before IOM Committee (Washington, D.C., June 6, 1980).

83. Connecticut Hospital Association, Extended Hospital Stay: A Serious Problem That's Growing Worse, Report No. 2 (CHA: January 6, 1980); Karen Dumbaugh and Robert Mackler, Report on Patients in Massachusetts Hospitals Awaiting Placement into Long Term Care (Massachusetts Hospital Association, 1979); National Capital Medical Foundation, Inappropriate Use of District Hospitals, 1978 (Washingon, D.C.: NCMF, 1978); New York Statewide Professional Standards Review Council, Inc., "Report on a Statewide Survey of Patients Awaiting Placement for Alternative Care Facilities in New York State, June 1979," press release (New York, 1979).

84. T. Willemain, E. Bishop, and A. Plough, "The Nursing Home 'Level of Care' Problem," University Health Policy Consortium (Waltham, MA: Brandeis University, 1980) p. 8.

85. Congressional Budget Office, Long Term Care for The Elderly and Disabled (Washington, D.C.: Government Printing Office, 1977) p. x.

86. U.S. General Accounting Office, p. 19.

5

LEGAL MECHANISMS FOR CIVIL RIGHTS ENFORCEMENT

There is a general lack of awareness of civil rights issues in health care, but a framework of laws exists within which disparities that may be due to discrimination can be addressed. This chapter describes three legal bases for actions against racial/ethnic discrimination in health care delivery--Title VI of the Civil Rights Act, the health planning legislation, and the Hill-Burton Act for facilities construction.

This chapter also briefly reviews the enforcement of existing civil rights legislation. The review suggests that, while existing law has limitations, the lack of effective enforcement of existing laws has been a major impediment to defining more clearly the scope and nature of civil rights in health care. Federal agencies have been authorized, and in some cases mandated, to collect data, identify relevant issues, and establish and enforce policies regarding discrimination in the delivery of health services. However, neither the enforcement program for Title VI, the major vehicle for civil rights enforcement in health care, nor the activities carried out under the federal health planning program have provided a basic description of relevant problems. Available enforcement mechanisms have received only limited use and development, and their potential influence has just begun to be felt.

The first serious attempts to apply civil rights law to the delivery of health services are still under way, and their consequences are uncertain. The specific legal meaning of discrimination in the health care context will grow out of such cases as are described in this chapter. It should be emphasized that civil rights as a concept is not "set"; the law is an evolving process. Legal cases both reflect and determine societal concensus as to what is discrimination. Legal issues and cases are presented in this chapter not only to show the present status of civil rights activities in health care but also to stimulate wider debate that may help clarify many issues and questions.

This chapter does not attempt to summarize or catalog all relevant laws or the manner in which they are or could be enforced, and it does not specifically extend the analysis of the previous chapter regarding handicapped persons. It describes the laws that are likely to be the major bases for legal challenges to discrimination, particularly on the basis of race or ethnicity, in the forseeable future.

OVERVIEW OF CIVIL RIGHTS LAWS

Since the civil rights litigation of the 1950s and 1960s and the Supreme Court's abandonment of the "separate but equal" interpretation of the Equal Protection Clause of the Fourteenth Amendment, it has been established that the federal constitution prohibits discrimination by the government on the basis of race. This constitutional prohibition has been supplemented and extended through federal and state legislative and administrative enactments prohibiting racial discrimination by recipients of federal funds, by government contractors, by most private and public employers, in public accommodations, and in many other activities. Although wholly private activities are exempt from the proscription of the federal constitution, Congress or state legislatures under various jurisdictional bases can prohibit racial discrimination in many private activities. A variety of legislatively and administratively established prohibitions apply to the delivery of health care by both public and private providers and include legislation enacted by Congress and some states in the last decade prohibiting discrimination on the basis of sex, age, or handicap.

TITLE VI OF THE CIVIL RIGHTS ACT OF 1964

The Civil Rights Act of 1964[1] established the authority for a variety of federal governmental initiatives to end discrimination in voting, public accommodations, education, and nearly all other activities under federal jurisdiction. Title VI of that act prohibited racial discrimination by recipients of federal financial assistance:

> No person in the United States shall, on the ground of race, color or national origin, be excluded from participation in, be denied the benefits of, or be subjected to discrimination under any program or activity receiving federal financial assistance.

Title VI also required federal agencies to implement this policy in their programs by issuing regulations and terminating federal assistance in the event of failure to comply with Title VI.[2] In 1965 the Department of Health, Education, and Welfare (DHEW) issued its first set of interpretative regulations that gave substance to the Title VI prohibition on discrimination by recipients of departmental funds.[3] These were amended in 1973 and have not been revised again. (See Appendix B for the full text of the substantive portion of the regulations.)

Although activities in the health sector largely took a back seat to questions of discrimination in education, the potential implications of civil rights activities in health care are broad. The regulations interpret Title VI to prohibit not only the denial of services or benefits on the basis of race, color, or national origin, but also to prohibit any form of differential or segregated treatment. They further prohibit discrimination in a variety of related contexts (such as site location and selection of membership for boards) and make it clear that the jurisdictional reach of Title VI goes beyond overt acts of discrimination:

> A recipient . . . may not, directly or through contractual or other agreements, utilize criteria or methods of administration which have the effect of subjecting individuals to discrimination.[4]

However, because the regulations were generalized for all of DHEW, they give little indication of how they would apply to the specific circumstances of health care delivery. They include no specific reference to the obligations of health care providers. Specific "guidelines" for compliance by hospitals and nursing homes were issued in 1969 in the form of letters executed by the Director of the Office for Civil Rights (OCR).[5] The guidelines (Appendix C) provide the major specific federal interpretation of the Title VI responsibilities of health care providers. They cover such matters as the meaning of the Title VI prohibition on discrimination in admission procedures, room assignments, referral arrangements, and staff privileges in hospitals and nursing homes. In addition, the hospital and nursing home guidelines indicate that underutilization by minorities is itself a source of concern. As stated in the hospital guidelines:

> Where there is a significant variation between the racial composition of the patient census and available population census data for the service area or potential service area, the hospital has a responsibility to determine the reason for such variation and to take whatever action may be necessary to correct any discrimination.[6]

This guideline does not define discrimination. Nor does it recognize that defining service areas raises a variety of methodological and political problems. For example, the extent of statistical under-representation may be heavily influenced by where the boundaries of service areas are drawn, as well as by what data and methods of estimation are used.

More recently, the OCR drafted compliance guidelines for other recipients of health-related funds (for example, state Medicaid agencies, health planning agencies, mental health centers), but these have never received clearance by all parts of the department and been made final. Thus, the 1969 guidelines are the only available official interpretation of Title VI in the health care context.

This lack of policy specification and clarification has hampered enforcement efforts. For example, the Title VI responsibilities of state and local planning agencies have never been clear. Nor has OCR formally determined whether private physicians who participate in Medicare or Medicaid have responsibilities under Title VI. Even with regard to hospitals and nursing homes, the guidelines do not specify the data to be used to monitor compliance, the procedures to be used for monitoring and enforcement activities, or the remedies that will be sought when discrimination is identified.

The size and organization of OCR also has limited Title VI enforcement.[7] Since 1968 the primary responsibility for enforcement of civil rights laws within DHEW (and later DHHS) has rested with a separate OCR in the Office of the Secretary. As of January 1980 (prior to the creation of the Department of Education from the old DHEW), OCR was budgeted for a staff of 1,700, 450 in Washington and the remainder in the 12 regional offices, to cover all aspects of civil rights monitoring and enforcement in DHEW programs.[8] But the investigative staff numbered only about 600 in the regional offices. However, OCR attorneys have been assisted by attorneys from the DHEW Office of General Counsel and by Justice Department attorneys when disputes required formal adjudication. OCR can also occasionally "borrow" personnel from other programs and hire outside consultants as the budget permits.

OCR has no direct supervisory or mandatory control over any program activities or program staff within the department. OCR activities and decisions affecting individual programs are negotiated by OCR staff with personnel from the various programs, and the resolution of conflicts between OCR and program staff requires intervention by the Office of the Secretary.[9]

As has been stated, most of the work of OCR heretofore has been on issues in education; prior to 1980, as little as 10 percent of OCR's staff and resources were committed to health or welfare issues. However, in April 1980, following the creation of the new Department of Education and the consolidation of the remaining DHEW programs into the DHHS, only about two-thirds of the OCR staff moved to the new department.[10] The one-third of the previous OCR staff forming the OCR in DHHS represents a substantial increase in the resources available for civil rights activities in health and welfare.

Even before the division into the two departments, however, OCR was showing increased concern with civil rights issues in health and welfare, in part as a result of pressure from private advocacy groups that successfully brought suit to force increased enforcement activities with regard to health care providers.[11] The increased activity is evident, for example, in a projection by the Director of OCR of Title VI activities for fiscal year 1981, which included investigation of all civil rights complaints against health facilities plus more than 250 compliance reviews of hospitals, nursing homes, and state health-related agencies.[12] In addition, OCR undertook a large Title VI compliance survey of hospitals in late 1980. These activities prescribe an ambitious agenda for OCR, particularly in light of its limited experience in health issues.

Although OCR's plans include a large number of compliance reviews (that is, on-site evaluations of the compliance of an agency or facility with the requirements of Title VI) of hospitals, nursing homes, and other recipients of health-related DHHS funds, few have been undertaken in the past, and no substantive guidelines or procedures for compliance assessment of any of these institutions exist in other than draft form. Historically, OCR has relied heavily on individual complaints to direct its enforcement efforts. Until very recently, however, there have been few Title VI complaints filed against health care providers or other health-related institutions. Consequently, OCR has conducted few individual investigations of health care providers.[13]

However, the number of complaints alleging discrimination in health services has markedly increased in the past three or four years.[14] Virtually all of the recent health-related investigations of OCR have been the product of privately initiated lawsuits or individual complaints. The New Orleans lawsuit, Cook v. Ochsner Foundation Hospital (summarized in Appendix E) is an example.

OCR has also been responsible for monitoring the Title VI compliance of all recipients of departmental funds. In the past, however, the compliance of health care providers has not been monitored on a comprehensive or periodic basis; the monitoring activities have been confined to the requirement that providers receiving federal funds execute (and periodically re-execute) assurances of non-discrimination.[15] No data on health services have regularly been collected for civil rights enforcement purposes, and data collected by statistical agencies (such as the National Center for Health Statistics) or for program monitoring have been of limited usefulness for identifying possible civil rights problems. Occasional studies of certain providers in localized geographic regions have been conducted under OCR auspices, and a one-day hospital inpatient census was conducted in 1969 and again in 1973 (with inconclusive results).[16] Health facilities are required to execute non-discrimination assurances as part of initial certification, and the policies of most nursing homes are reviewed as part of the recertification review for Medicare and Medicaid eligibilty, but no monitoring of actual services rendered has been done on either a sample or across-the-board basis.

In a related activity, for the past 10 years OCR has attempted to secure assurances from state agencies that they are not discriminating in the federal health and welfare programs they administer and that they are assessing the compliance of recipient institutions, including health care providers.[17] Although many regional OCR offices devote substantial time and effort to state agency compliance review, apparently little useful data collection or monitoring of health care providers has resulted.

OTHER APPROACHES TO CIVIL RIGHTS ENFORCEMENT

Although direct application of Title VI is the primary vehicle for federal enforcement of civil rights in health care, some of the same objectives may also be pursued through other administrative activities, including the health planning and Hill-Burton programs.

The Health Planning Program

The 1974 National Health Planning Resources Development Act was not developed specifically as a response to issues arising in the health care of racial and ethnic minority groups. Nevertheless, the mandate of the planning agencies established by the act addresses several issues relevant to civil rights concerns. Planning agencies are responsible for developing plans that, among other things, assure that health services are available and accessible to all residents of the area. Thus, they must confront problems of unequal access to health care, the needs of medically underserved populations, and disparities in health status. These are issues that, in many parts of the country, pertain to disproportionate numbers of minority groups. However, for several reasons, which may include the limited authority and resources of planning agencies and the lack of consistent federal guidance regarding how civil rights concerns might appropriately be addressed by health planning agencies, the planning program has given only limited explicit attention to civil rights issues.[18]

In carrying out their responsibilities, health planning agencies are to consider civil rights as one factor in making decisions such as approving new services, facilities, and other capital expenditures, and reviewing the appropriateness of existing facilities. How that is to be done and how civil rights considerations are to be weighted relative to other social goals are not clear. Whether planning agencies are required under Title VI to modify or defer decisions where Title VI violations are alleged has been a matter of some controversy, as is shown by the New Orleans case described in Appendix E. The statutory scheme implies that services to minorities be considered along with a variety of other factors in health planning decisions. This implication can be seen in the statutory requirement for the development of federal guidelines that would "reflect the unique circumstances and needs of medically underserved populations," and for state health planning agencies to consider "the extent to which such proposed services will be accessible to all the residents of the area to be served by such services" in making certificate-of-need decisions.*

---

*In addition to the statutory language, the regulations recently proposed for planning agencies in administering state certificate of need programs would require specific consideration of the unmet needs of minorities.[19] If adopted, these regulations would require planning agencies, in making certificate of need decisions, to make written findings about the impact of the proposed service on minorities, including the extent to which racial minorities (and other underserved groups) are likely to have access to the proposed services and the past performance of the applicant in complying with Title VI and other civil rights laws.

Although there is little evidence that state and federal health planning agencies have brought civil rights considerations into planning activities, as a result of recent litigation and a developing interest within the agency, DHHS has recently begun to address the problems of racial minorities in the administration of health planning programs. First, the proposed regulations for the planning activites established by the planning act and Section 1122 of the Social Security Act explicitly require consideration of the health needs of minorities by state and local health planning agencies.[20] Second, DHHS has considered an interpretation of Title VI that would specifically require health care facilities and health planning agencies to provide and plan for services in a non-discriminatory manner.

The discussion to this point has concerned the authority of health planning agencies under their authorizing legislation. In addition, health planning agencies may also be required to address issues of access for minorities under the Civil Rights Act. Congress clearly intended Title VI of the Civil Rights Act of 1964 to prohibit discrimination in all federally funded programs. Although Title VI mandates all federal agencies to establish an administrative program to ensure that the prohibition incorporated into Title VI is enforced,[21] DHEW (and DHHS) has provided little procedural or substantive guidance about the requirements of Title VI compliance for state and local planning agencies funded through the planning program.

The potential impact of applying Title VI to health planning agencies and their decisions has been emphasized by recent controversies in New Orleans, Louisiana (Appendix E), and Wilmington, Delaware. These cases also illustrate the intractability of some of the problems that may arise.

In March 1976 the Wilmington Medical Center (WMC), claiming serious financial distress, proposed a major relocation of its facilities and services from a site in the heavily minority, inner city of Wilmington to a suburban site.[22] Since WMC participates in the Medicare and Medicaid programs, it sought "Sec. 1122 approval" for capital expenditures related to WMC's relocation plan (Plan Omega). Apparently without taking specific consideration of the impact on the minority population, the local and state health planning agencies reviewed the application and made favorable recommendations. DHEW gave final approval soon thereafter.

In September 1976, minority residents of Wilmington and several groups representing minorities filed suit in federal court charging that the removal of beds and services contemplated by the plan would deny them access to health care services which would be in violation of Title VI and its implementing regulations. DHEW and the local and state planning agencies, by virtue of the approval each had given the relocation plan under Section 1122, were charged with violating their obligations to enforce and comply with Title VI. The federal district court ordered DHEW's OCR to conduct an investigation.[23] OCR determined that implementation of Plan Omega would violate Title VI. However, after negotiations with WMC, OCR concluded that the potential violations could be eliminated by modifying the plan according to 12 remedial conditions, such as provision of transportation for residents of the inner city to the the new suburban site. WMC accepted the conditions and amended the original plan. The plaintiffs, however, were not satisfied with the settlement, and a series of new legal actions and appeals ensued.[24] The matter is still under appeal.

A legacy of the litigation is the original judicial recognition that a facility that closes or relocates services may violate Title VI and that private individuals have a right of action against both the facility and the government. The case is also important as the first recognition of the applicability to a health facility of the Title VI site relocation regulation (see Appendix B)--a regulation presumably written in contemplation of the relocation of educational facilities. Significant also was DHEW's position that the original relocation plan would violate Title VI if it had a "disparate effect" on minorities, even without a finding of intent to discriminate by the facility.

By finding that Plan Omega, as originally proposed, could violate Title VI, OCR established a link between Title VI and health facilities' ability to make such decisions, as well as a link between the planning/regulatory apparatus and civil rights concerns. Both links raised new and important legal and ethical questions in the organization of health services and health planning. OCR effectively held that Section 1122 reviews were inadequate if they failed to consider the site relocation regulation or other provisions of Title VI. By agreeing to make revisions in Plan Omega that would bring it into compliance with Title VI, OCR and WMC apparently agreed that the Title VI regulations applied to this type of decision. The Wilmington case suggests that an effective linkage of institutional planning, areawide health planning, and Title VI would require integration of civil rights considerations into the health planning process at an early stage. This would cover both the establishment of specific standards for determining compliance with Title VI and procedures for ensuring that those standards are adequately considered.

Recent events in New Orleans demonstrate other complexities of integrating Title VI considerations with institutional decision-making and health planning reviews at state and local levels. In the aftermath of Title VI litigation in New Orleans (see Appendix E), OCR attempted to require the Louisiana State Health Planning and Development Agency (LSHPDA) to deny or defer approval of Section 1122 applications from hospitals that had previously been found in non-compliance with Title VI.[25] However, the LSHPDA did not comply with OCR's deferral request,[26] arguing that DHEW's proper remedy was to take action terminating federal funds to hospitals that were not in compliance with Title VI. Subsequently, the Health Resources Administration (HRA) within DHEW granted final approval to the application. This placed DHEW in the position of having one of its agencies approving new federal funding to a hospital while another of its agencies was claiming that the approval must be deferred because of civil rights violations. To date, no steps have been taken to resolve this inconsistency. No clear and simple answer can be found in the authorizing statutes that will resolve the awkward departmental position of having two offices publicly taking contrary positions on an important social issue.

The controversies in Wilmington and New Orleans show a growing recognition of the possible application of civil rights to health planning. Regulations proposed in March 1980 could be a first step toward more explicit consideration of the needs of minorities in health planning decisions, although they do not specifically mention Title VI or establish an applicant facility's compliance with Title VI as a criterion of planning agency approval.

The Hill-Burton "Community Service" Obligation

Another program through which certain civil rights issues may be addressed is the Hill-Burton program and its successor legislation for facility construction in the National Health Planning and Resource Development Act of 1974. The assurances given by facilities that received funding under Hill-Burton provide a legal basis for addressing some of the problems described in Chapter 2, particularly those pertaining to refusals to accept Medicaid patients, a population that, in many areas of the country, contains disproportionate numbers of persons from racial and ethnic minorities.

The initial 1946 Hill-Burton program of federal grants for hospital construction represented more than financial assistance for hospitals and other health facilities.[27] It brought an unprecedented investment of federal funds into facility construction and an expansion of federal regulation into health care.[28] It also introduced planning on a nationwide basis. Participating states had to survey the need for health facilities and develop a state plan for health facility construction, establish programs for maintaining the quality and safety of funded projects, and meet a variety of other federal requirements in the administration of their survey and planning activities.[29] Similarly, funded projects had to meet relatively extensive federal requirements relating to construction standards, financial viability, and maintenance and operation of the funded facility and conform to the priorities established by their state plans.

The original legislation imposed on both the state agencies administering the program and the recipient facilities specific obligations to provide services to people who were unable to pay or were otherwise denied access to health facilities. These obligations have become the basis of legal challenges to hospital policies, such as refusal to accept Medicaid, that may establish significant barriers to many members of minority groups. The 1946 law required the development of state plans that, among other things would:

> provide for adequate hospital facilities for the people residing in a State, without discrimination on account of race, creed, or color, and for adequate hospital facilities for persons unable to pay therefore. Such regulation may require that before approval of any application for a hospital or addition to a hospital is recommended by a State agency, assurance shall be received

> by the State from the applicant that (1) such hospital or addition to a hospital will be made available to all persons residing in the territorial area of the applicant, without discrimination on account of race, creed, or color, but an exception shall be made in cases where separate hospital facilities are provided for separate population groups, if the plan makes equitable provision on the basis of need for facilities and services of like quality for each group; and (2) there will be made available in each such hospital or addition to a hospital a reasonable volume of hospital services to persons unable to pay therefore, but an exception shall be made if such a requirement is not feasible from a financial standpoint.[30]

These "charity care" obligations, as the requirements of this provision have been frequently labeled, ostensibly imposed two distinct obligations on recipient facilities: (1) to provide a reasonable volume of "uncompensated services" and (2) to be available to all residents without discrimination, generally referred to as the "community service" obligation. These obligations were an integral part of the original legislative scheme reflected in the declaration of purposes and throughout the other provisions of the original legislation. The language of the original "charity care" obligations was specifically added to the legislation as part of a political compromise to ensure the support of congressional liberals.[31] As the Hill-Burton legislation was amended to include new funding mechanisms and additional categories of funding recipients, Congress continued to re-enact these obligations as preconditions to funding. Even when the program was effectively terminated in 1974 by the National Health Planning and Resources Development Act, the successor federal program attached similar conditions to receipt of funds under the facility construction program authorized by the new legislation.[32] The 1974 legislation, while essentially replacing the Hill-Burton program, explicitly required DHEW to monitor and enforce the uncompensated service and community service obligations of recipients of funds under the Hill-Burton programs and the new program.[33] Further, institutions that had benefited from Hill-Burton continued to carry the obligation.

Until the early 1970s when several consumer-initiated lawsuits forced DHEW to give more than *pro forma* recognition to the matter, the statutory obligations were given no further specification in program regulations or guidelines and, as was later documented in hearings, the obligations were generally ignored by both recipient facilities, DHEW, and state Hill-Burton agencies.[34] To date, the obligation to provide a specific volume of uncompensated service has been the object of more attention than the community service obligation, although this may change in the future.

In 1972, under pressure from the courts, DHEW issued the first set of interpretive regulations specifying the meaning of the uncompensated service obligation and outlining a program that relied heavily on the state Hill-Burton agencies for monitoring compliance by Hill-Burton facilities.[35] Subsequent litigation by private consumer groups again attacked the adequacy of these efforts, and resulted in further amendments to the uncompensated services regulations in 1975.[36] After 1974 health planning legislation effectively mandated increased federal enforcement efforts, extensive federal hearings were held in 1978, and additional federal regulations interpreting the charity care obligations were issued in 1979.[37] Among other things, these new regulations committed DHEW to more rigorous enforcement of the uncompensated service obligation and defined more specifically the meaning of uncompensated service. However, because of a variety of problems surrounding the concept of uncompensated services, this aspect of the Hill-Burton obligations is a continuing source of controversy.

The second Hill-Burton obligation--that recipient facilities be available to all--has, until recently, received less attention than the uncompensated services provisions, even from the consumer advocacy groups responsible for the Hill-Burton "charity care" lawsuits. To be sure, the original legislatively mandated obligation is only a general policy statement, and even as a policy statement it is subject to two very different interpretations. Narrowly interpreted, it bans discrimination on the basis of race, creed, or color. On the other hand, the mandate to "provide hospital facilities for the people residing in a State, without discrimination on account of race, creed, or color," can be read to require open access to all people who need (and presumably who can pay) for the services of the facility. The implications of such a statement of policy can be far-reaching.

Ironically, the first meaningful interpretation of the "community service" obligation came from a federal court decision that invalidated a portion of the statutory language that created the charity care obligations. Relying on the Hill-Burton language that allowed a "separate but equal" exception to the prohibition of racial discrimination, the Public Health Service (and later DHEW) had, during the first two decades of the program, given Hill-Burton grants to a number of facilities that had open and official policies of racial discrimination.[38] In 1963 the Court of Appeals in Simkins v. Moses H. Cone Memorial Hospital ruled that the relevant portions of the federal statute and related regulations permitting this discriminatory practice were unconstitutional.[39]

As a result of this decision, when Congress recodified and expanded the Hill-Burton program in 1964, the provision establishing the "charity care" obligation was amended, modifying the "community service" language and omitting the "separate but equal" exception:

> (f) That the State plan shall provide for adequate hospitals, and other facilities for which aid under this part is available, for all persons residing in the State, and adequate hospitals (and such other facilities) to furnish needed services for persons unable to pay therefore. Such regulations may also require that before approval of an application for a project is recommended by

> a State agency to the Surgeon General for approval under this part, assurance shall be received by the State from the applicant that (1) the facility or portion thereof to be constructed or modernized will be made available to all persons residing in the territorial area of the applicant; and (2) there will be made available in the facility or portion thereof to be constructed or modernized a reasonable volume of services to persons unable to pay therefore, but an exception shall be made if such a requirement is not feasible from a financial viewpoint.[40]

The federal program regulations issued in 1964 following the statutory amendment required that recipient facilities comply with the community service obligation and gave a general interpretation of its meaning, but they gave little indication that DHEW was committed to its enforcement.[41] The regulations did, however, indicate that in order to comply with the statute, funded facilities both must not discriminate on the basis of race, creed, color, or national origin and must furnish a "community service"--the first use of that particular term to specify the obligation of Hill-Burton facilities.[42] "Community service," as defined by the 1964 regulations, meant that (1) the services furnished are available to the general public or (2) admission is limited only on the basis of age, medical indigency, or type or kind of mental or medical disability." Thus, DHEW's view was that the statutory amendment had left the essential obligation unchanged, except for the elimination of the separate-but-equal exception. As with earlier "charity care" regulations, however, the 1964 regulations included no reference to monitoring or enforcement of the obligations.

In 1974, under court order, DHEW issued regulations further interpreting "community service" to require recipients to participate in Medicare and Medicaid and to "take such steps as necessary" to ensure that Medicare and Medicaid patients were admitted without discrimination.[43] But while the regulations clarified the meaning of the statutory term "available to all" and the term "community service" as used in the 1964 regulations, the 1974 regulations did not impose explicit standards for assessing compliance with the requirements. State Hill-Burton agencies were given almost total discretion to develop methods for evaluating and enforcing the obligations.

In 1979, DHEW issued new charity care regulations (Appendix D) for both Hill-Burton facilities and facilities funded under the newer health facility construction program authorized by the 1974 legislation. In these regulations the community service obligation was made much more specific.[44] The essential mandate of these regulations was to specify that the community service assurance required Hill-Burton facilities to be open to all residents of a facility's service area who are (1) able to pay and (2) in need of the services provided by the facility.[45] Furthermore, the regulations require recipient facilities to provide emergency services to all residents, regardless of ability to pay, and to discharge or transfer a person after rendering emergency services only after making a determination that doing so would not result in a substantial risk to the individual.[46] The regulations also explicitly require the recipient to accept Medicaid and Medicare patients and implicitly require the facility to accept all third-party payment.

In addition to these substantive requirements, the regulations also define certain practices as presumptively in violation of the community service obligation and explicitly list certain practices that may have to be modified if they result in patients being excluded from receiving care. For example, a policy of admitting only persons who have a physician on the facility's medical staff may have the effect of preventing a facility from meeting its obligation to be generally available to the community.[47]

These regulations have important implications for minorities and others who traditionally have had problems gaining access to health care. The community service obligation is imposed in perpetuity, unlike the uncompensated service obligation, which expires 20 years after the receipt of Hill-Burton funds.[48] Furthermore, the community service obligation requires participation in Medicaid, not as a remedial requirement, but as a substantive requirement imposed on all Hill-Burton facilities. The regulations define such particiption not just as being certified as an eligible Medicaid provider, but as providing service to a representative portion of the Medicaid population. Thus, whether discrimination against minorities is an intended or unintended consequence of discrimination against Medicaid and other governmental program recipients, these regulations provide a legal device by which the problem can be addressed.

These regulations may also indirectly impose obligations on private physicians who are members of the medical staff of a Hill-Burton hospital, at least to the extent that a physician's activities can be causally linked to the compliance of the facility.[49] This might arise, for example, in a situation in which hospitals admit only patients of staff physicians and staff physicians refuse to accept Medicaid patients.

Thus, the community service regulations may provide a basis for eliminating some practices that have a disparate effect on minorities in situations where the application of Title VI may not be clearly defined. The validity and enforcement of the new Hill-Burton regulations has already been challenged by health providers.[50] Thus far, the courts have upheld their validity, but it will be many years before the regulations will have been fully applied and tested before the courts.

How DHHS will enforce the community service regulations remains to be seen. After the May 1979 regulations were issued, DHEW held workshops for consumers and providers to explain DHEW enforcement plans. The materials produced for these workshops indicated that a plan of enforcement would not be implemented immediately and would emphasize compliance with the uncompensated service, rather than the community service obligation.[51] The regulations' relevance to civil rights concerns, however, is reinforced by the increased involvement of the OCR in their enforcement. In January 1980 the OCR entered into an agreement with the Public Health Service to assume some departmental responsibility for enforcement of the community service obligation. In August 1980 the Secretary of DHHS decided to give full responsibility to OCR, although that decision was not immediately implemented.

CONCLUSIONS

This review of selected civil rights legal issues in health care leads the committee to conclude that there have been serious limitations in enforcement and monitoring. In particular, there has been little effective monitoring of civil rights compliance, in part because the concept of compliance has been ill-defined and, thus, appropriate measures of compliance have not been determined. Existing regulations are vague when applied to health services and institutions. There is also a lack of clarity in the definition of the role of planning agencies in implementing Title VI.

Interest in civil rights in health care has grown in recent years, and the creation of the DHHS brought about a significant increase in resources available for civil rights enforcement in health. However, an examination of recent enforcement efforts and testimony before the committee forcefully demonstrates that there is no consensus on a conceptual framework for evaluating "compliance" by health care providers, and, until further specifications can be made of what constitutes civil rights noncompliance by providers, monitoring efforts will be unfocused.

Although the hospital and nursing home guidelines issued by OCR in 1969 have shortcomings, their usefulness has been repeatedly noted by agency staff and representatives of civil rights groups. There is a clear need, however, for further clarification and specification of the requirements of Title VI and Section 504 in health care. OCR's recent investigations have been made on an *ad hoc*, *ex post facto* basis. Data needs were defined in the course of the investigation, and no criteria were available against which compliance could be judged. More stable civil rights enforcement efforts require codification of assumptions and procedures. Several policies have emerged out of civil rights enforcement efforts in recent years that should be more widely debated and, perhaps, codified in regulations or guidelines. Examples include the conclusions incident to the recent hospital relocation investigation in Wilmington, Delaware, regarding physical access to health services, the availability of transportation, and the problems inherent in duplication of services--particularly as these affect members of minority and handicapped groups; the remedial requirements developed in the New Orleans investigation (Appendix E) for hospitals found in noncompliance with Title VI; and the OCR positions (implied by the 1969 guidelines) on apparent underutilization of health services by minorities and on the issue of whether a showing of *intent* to discriminate is a necessary requisite of a finding that discrimination is, in fact, occurring.

In addition, the committee has noted a number of circumstances in which existing policies are confusing or ambiguous and that warrant specific interpretation and clarification:

- The Title VI responsibilities of health planning agencies, including any requirements that civil rights be built into the plans and decisions of state and local planning agencies, and the extent of their discretionary authority to give priority to providers that engage in affirmative action.
- The responsibities of hospitals and other facilities serving substantial numbers of non-English speaking people (such as requirements for interpreters or translations of basic documents such as patient consent forms).
- The scope and nature of Title VI responsibilities of health facilities that plan to close or convert their services.
- The scope and nature of responsibilities of health providers and health planning agencies under Section 504 of the Rehabilitation Act.

The ambiguities in the definitions of discrimination in health cannot, however, be completely "solved" by administrative remedies. In the future, as in the past, the impact of OCR enforcement efforts under Title VI and Section 504 will depend, in large part, on the judicial interpretation of whether a discriminatory effect, without a showing of discriminatory intent, constitutes a legal violation. If the legal promise of non-discrimination is to be defined and enforced in practical terms in the health area, it is essential to decide whether or not the "effects" approach--that is, concern about policies or practices that have racially disparate effects, whatever their intent--of the existing guidelines is to be taken seriously or, indeed, whether it will even be retained.

The guidelines issued by OCR in 1969 delineate standards on which initial judgments can be made as to whether there is a cause for concern about racially disparate effects, and they set out the nature of the justification that may constitute acceptable explanations for these effects. The committee recommends that 1969 guidelines be proposed as formal regulations for DHHS, either in their present form or in a revised version that retains the essential "effects" approach to defining violations of Title VI. While the 1969 guidelines are hardly the final word on defining discrimination in health care, they provide a useful place to begin the process of debate, consensus, definition, and enforcement of civil rights in the health arena. Formal proposal in the Federal Register would not only make an important statement about the commitment of DHHS to the enforcement of civil rights, but would also provide the occasion for public comment by all concerned parties that would itself prompt further refinement of basic principles.

Certain existing *de facto* policies should also be reconsidered. For example, OCR has historically distinguished between access and quality, claiming that, under Title VI, evaluations can be made of admissions to available services but not of the adequacy of the service rendered. This notion, which follows civil rights approaches in education, has consequences for the data collected and procedures followed in compliance reviews. While quality of medical care in its strictest sense may be impossible to assess in the context of Title VI reviews, some surrogate measures of quality, such as length of stay or readmission rates, might be useful indicators of problem areas that need more focused investigation. Quality assurance efforts of many types are being undertaken throughout the country, in many cases by federally funded professional standards review organizations (PSROs). However, the potential usefulness of these efforts for identifying inappropriate racial and ethnic differences in health care has been largely untapped.

The most widely used measures of civil rights compliance are aggregate measures of admissions to institutional providers itemized by racial/ethnic categories. Measures of services to those with handicaps are even more rudimentary, because few basic data are available on medical needs and use of services by handicapped persons. The committee found that there are serious shortcomings in data both for assessing compliance by health care providers and for assessing more generally overall problems in the health services provided to and/or needed by minorities and the handicapped. Such data are prerequisites to enforcement activities under present legal obligations and to the continuing process of definition as to what disparities are to be regarded as unreasonable or illegitimate in terms of civil rights laws.

The committee regards as essential the development within OCR of greater technical expertise in health-related data analysis. OCR should work with existing data-collection agencies, such as the National Center for Health Statistics, to specify and obtain data needed for pursuit of OCR's responsibilities. Similarly, closer cooperation between OCR and the Health Care Financing Administration can lead to development of measures and indicators that will help focus compliance review activities. OCR should also consider the possible usefulness for civil rights activities of data collected by other agencies in DHHS and recommend changes needed to facilitate enforcement procedures.

The committee suggests that the OCR inventory available indicators and measures of civil rights compliance, including available and potential sources of data. Much of the information contained in this report pertains to such an inventory.

However, data collection is a hollow exercise, unless further specification can be made of what constitutes civil rights noncompliance by health care providers. Data collection and analysis are useless as compliance vehicles unless they are guided by informed judgments about possible explanations for disparities in the provision of services. This report suggests some of the complexities that must be faced in reaching such judgments and suggests some materials on which they might be made.

In addition, decisions must be made about allocation of effort among various kinds of enforcement activities. OCR has announced its intention to undertake several hundred compliance reviews of health care institutions each year. Because of limited OCR resources, this may result in less attention to individual complaints. Furthermore, given the present state of knowledge about the reasons for racial/ethnic disparities in health status and use of services, an emphasis on compliance reviews suggests unwarranted certainty that specific elements of discrimination can be identified and measured. On the other hand, while an emphasis on complaint investigation might lead to testing and refinement of what constitutes unlawful discrimination in health care activities, it may also dissipate energies as many complaints are found to lack merit. The implications of these different approaches deserve careful consideration in establishing policies for the OCR.

Another issue concerns the proper scope of compliance reviews, which may focus on either individual institutions or geographic areas. Some striking racial/ethnic patterns become evident only when an investigation goes beyond a particular institution and considers the use of services in, for example, an entire metropolitan area. However, recent civil rights investigations in New Orleans and Wilmington show that broad compliance reviews require a major commitment of OCR resources. Although it may be possible to husband resources by limiting the issues to be assessed in a compliance review and by relying wherever possible on data collected for other purposes (for example, by PSROs), OCR's present staffing appears to be inadequate to conduct major compliance reviews of a large number of institutions.

Besides civil rights enforcement *per se*, the enforcement of the community service and equal access obligations of Hill-Burton facilities could have an important impact on alleviating some circumstances that have led to the unequal treatment of minorities by institutional health care providers.

The juncture of civil rights and health planning, which involves different agencies within DHHS, raises the need for coordination so that policies will be coherent and consistent. For example, clarification is needed regarding OCR's authority to direct planning agencies to defer approval of proposals pending completion of a fund termination hearing. The kinds of enforcement activities now being contemplated, such as compliance reviews of major institutions, require more internal specification within DHHS of lines of authority and operating procedures, in addition to the delineation of substantive policy.

Finally, because access to health facilities is often dependent upon access to, and the behavior of, private physicians, the committee recommends that OCR reconsider the informal policy under which private practitioners have been exempted from Title VI and related compliance requirements, even if they receive payments under Part B of Medicare.

Existing civil rights concerns are largely encapsulated in OCR and administered in a way that allow other DHEW/DHHS programs to hold OCR, and its concerns, at arms length. Yet virtually all monitoring and enforcement activities eventually rely on some degree of cooperation between OCR and other DHHS programs, from health planning to Medicare. If effective efforts are to be made to pursue civil rights in health services--and the committee strongly believes that such efforts should be made--a clear commitment to do so is needed from agency leadership. This commitment is particularly important because the difficulties of definition, the ambiguities in policies, and the differences of opinion that must be taken into account in approaching questions of disparities in the current health system, over and above overt discrimination on the basis of handicap or race. Without such commitment, the enforcement of civil rights laws in the context of health care delivery may well continue to be haunted by administrative inconsistencies that are apparent to the courts, reviewing bodies, and the recipients themselves. The committee urges the Secretary of DHHS to resolve the present administrative ambiguities about civil rights within the agency, to make plain the commitment to the enforcement of the law's guarantees of non-discrimination, and to require all components of DHHS to cooperate with OCR in making these ideals a reality.

REFERENCES

1. Pub. L. No. 88-352, 78 Stat. 240 (1964).
2. Pub. L. No. 88-352, Title VI, §601-602, 78 Stat. 252-3 (1964), codified at 42 U.S.C. §2000d-2000d-1 (1978 Supp.). The Title VI directive to federal agencies regarding enforcement of the policy set forth in Title VI is as follows:

    Each federal department and agency which is empowered to extend federal financial assistance to any program of activity, by way of grant, loan, or contract other than a contract of insurance of guaranty, is authorized and directed to effectuate the provisions of section 2000d of this title with respect to such program activity by issuing rules, regulations, or orders of general applicability which shall be consistent with achievement of the objectives of the statute authorizing the financial assistance in connection with which the action is taken. No such rule, regulation, or order shall become effective unless and until approved by the President. Compliance with any requirement adopted pursuant to this section may be effected (1) by the termination of or refusal to grant or to continue assistance under such program or activity to any recipient as to whom there has been an express finding on the record, after opportunity for hearing, of a failure to comply with such requirement, but such termination or refusal shall be limited to the particular political entity, or part thereof, or other recipient as to whom such a finding has been made and, shall be limited in its effect to the particular program, or part thereof, in which such noncompliance has been so found, or (2) by any other measure authorized by law. Provided, however, that no such action shall be taken until the department or agency concerned has advised the appropriate person or persons of the failure to comply with the requirement and has determined that compliance cannot be secured by voluntary means. In the case of any action terminating, or refusing to grant or continue, assistance because of failure to comply with a requirement imposed pursuant to this section, the head of the federal department or agency shall file with the committees of the House and Senate having legislative jurisdiction over the program or activity involved a full written report of the circumstances and the grounds for such action. No such action shall become effective until thirty days have elapsed after the filing of such report.

3. 30 Federal Register 35 (1965), establishing 45 C.F.R. §80 et seq.
4. 45 C.F.R. §80.3(b)(2) (1979).
5. OCR, DHEW, Guidelines for Compliance of Nursing Homes and Similar Facilities With Title VI of the Civil Rights Act of 1964; Guidelines for Compliance of Hospitals With Title VI of the Civil Rights Act of 1964; (issued in revised form November 1969).
6. Guidelines for Compliance of Hospitals, p. 2.
7. Kenneth Wing, "Title VI and Health Facilities: Forms Without Substance," 30 Hastings Law Journal 137 (1978).
8. OCR, DHEW Annual Operating Plan for Fiscal Year 1980, 44 Federal Register 76864 (1979).
9. For example, see the conflict that developed between OCR and the Public Health Service as described later in this chapter.
10. OCR, DHEW, "Final Background Paper on Health Care and Civil Rights," (presented to the U.S. Civil Rights Commission April 1980).
11. See discussion in 44 Federal Register 45255 (1979).
12. OCR, DHEW Final Background Paper . . ., p. 8.
13. Wing, pp. 172-3.
14. 44 Federal Register 76864, 76865 (1979).
15. Wing, pp. 161-5.
16. Ibid., p. 175.
17. Ibid., p. 168.
18. For a broad assessment of health planning program, see Institute of Medicine, Health Planning in the United States: Issues in Guideline Development, (Washington, D.C.: National Academy of Sciences, 1980), and Harry P. Cain and Helen N. Darling, "Health Planning in the United States: Where We Stand Today," Health Policy and Education 1 (1979) pp. 5-25.
19. See S. Newman, "Equal Access to Health Care: Health Planning Agencies' Obligations," 5 Health Law Project Library Bulletin 1 (July 1980).
20. 45 Federal Register 20026 (1980).
21. 42 U.S.C. §2000d-1 (1979).
22. For background of this proposal and the ensuing litigation, see National Association for the Advancement of Colored People et al. v. The Wilmington Medical Center, Inc. et al., Civ. Action No. 83-1893 (3d Cir. 1980).

23. 426 F. Supp. 919 (D. Del. 1977).
24. 453 F. Supp. 280 (D. Del. 1978). The decision was appealed to the Third Circuit Court of Appeals, 599 F.2d 124 (3d Cir. 1979), which ordered a new trial in which the district court again ruled that the plan did not violate Title VI. Judgment and order of the District Court for the District of Delaware dated May 13, 1980.
25. David S. Tatel, Director, Office for Civil Rights, letter to Hamilton V. Reid, Executive Director, Southern Baptist Hospital, May 24, 1978.
26. David S. Tatel, Director, Office for Civil Rights, letter to Ronald F. Falgout, Chief Administrative Officer, Louisiana State Health Planning and Development Agency, August 22, 1978.
27. Pub. L. No. 79-725, 60 Stat. 1041 (1946).
28. Wing and Craige, "Health Care Regulation: The Dilemma of a Partially Developed Public Policy," 57 North Carolina Law Review 1165, 1187 (1979).
29. See generally Public Health Service Act §612, 622, and 623, as amended by Pub. L. No. 79-725, §2, 60 Stat. 1041 (1946). cf. 42 U.S.C. §291(c)-(d) (1974).
30. Public Health Service Act §622(f) as amended by Pub. L. No. 79-725, §2, 60 Stat. 1041 (1946).
31. M. Rose, "Federal Regulation or Services to the Poor Under the Hill-Burton Act: Realities and Pitfalls," 70 Northwestern University Law Review 168 (1975).
32. Public Health Service Act §1602(5), as amended by Pub. L. No. 93-641, §4, 88 Stat. 2259 (1975), adding 42 U.S.C. §300-1(5) (1974-78 Supp.).
33. Public Health Service Act §1602(6) as amended by Pub. L. No. 93-641, §4, 88 Stat. 2259 (1975), adding 42 U.S.C. §3000-1(6) (1974-78 Supp.).
34. Rose, p. 169.
35. 37 Federal Register 14719, amending 42 C.F.R. §53.111-113 (1972).
36. 40 Federal Register 46203 (1975).
37. 44 Federal Register 29372 (1979).
38. Wing, pp. 144-5.
39. 323 F.2d 959 (4th Cir. 1963), cert. denied, 376 U.S. 793 (1964).
40. Public Health Service Act §603(e), as amended by Pub. L. No. 88-443, §3, 78 Stat. 451 (1964).
41. Rose, p. 169.
42. 29 Federal Register 16298, amending 42 C.F.R. §111-113 (1964).
43. 39 Federal Register 31767 (1974).
44. 44 Federal Register 29372 (1979), adding a new 42 C.F.R. part 124.
45. 42 C.F.R. §124.603(a) (1979).
46. 42 C.F.R. §124.603(b) (1979).
47. 42 C.F.R. §124.603(c) (1979).
48. 42 C.F.R. §124.603(d)(1) (1979).
49. cf. 42 C.F.R. §124.601 (1979) with 42 C.F.R. §501 (1979).
50. American Hospital Association v. Harris, Civ. Action No. 79c 2669 (N.D. Ill. 1980).
51. PHS, DHEW, Uncompensated Care and Community Service Obligations Compliance Standards Manual for Facility Personnel, (Washington, D.C.: Government Printing Office, 1980).

APPENDIX A

RACIAL PATTERNS WITHIN MEDICARE AND MEDICAID

An examination of racial/ethnic patterns in the use of medical services within the Medicare and Medicaid programs is important for two reasons. First, since these programs involve massive amounts of federal funds, they are a major arena for concerns that may arise under Title VI of the Civil Rights Act. Secondly, since both ability to pay and source of payment may affect people's ability to obtain medical care, an examination of situations in which these factors do not vary will help illuminate the effect of racial and ethnic factors themselves. Thus, an examination of patterns of medical care within the Medicare and Medicaid programs will help demonstrate whether minority group members face disproportionate barriers in seeking medical care.

Medicare is the federal health insurance for the aged and certain disabled persons. The eligibility requirements and benefit structure are the same throughout the country and apply without regard to income or assets. Medicare involves two types of insurance benefits. Part A covers inpatient hospital care, post-hospital extended care, and post-hospital home health care and is automatically provided to anyone eligible for Social Security payments. Part B covers physicians and related services and is financed in part by monthly premiums paid by beneficiaries. In fiscal year 1978, about 23 million persons (over 95 percent of the elderly) were eligible for Part A coverage, and most (98 percent of whites and 96 percent of nonwhites in 1976) of these were also covered under Part B.[1]

Racial Trends Within Medicare. In an analysis of 1968 Medicare data, Davis explored whether aged Medicare enrollees used benefits equally, regardless of race, income, or place of residence.[2] She found expenditures per black enrollee under Medicare were smaller than expenditures per white enrollee. This difference was due to the fact that a smaller proportion of blacks than whites received benefits under the program. (Reimbursement amounts per person served, however, were essentially equal across racial groups.) The disadvantage of blacks was most severe for physician services and extended care facilities, and was most pronounced in the South. Davis's findings raised concerns about relative entitlements, by race, within the Medicare program in its early years.

Ruther and Dobson have examined more recent (1976) Medicare data to see whether the racial differences reported by Davis have persisted.[3] Their conclusions were, that although racial disparities still existed, they had decreased in the period between 1967 and 1976. Their data for those two years, presented in terms of the ratio of whites to nonwhites receiving various types of services, are shown in Table 22.

Although the racial differences have generally diminished, whites still use inpatient hospital services and physician services under Medicare at somewhat higher rates than do nonwhites. The white use of skilled nursing facilities under Medicare is still much higher than that of nonwhites. Given that black health status is, on average, lower than white health status, these patterns seem anomalous. On the other hand, Table 22 also shows that nonwhites are more likely to make use of outpatient departments (perhaps reflecting a lack of access to private physicians) and home health agencies.

In sum, even though racial differences have diminished in the Medicare program, available data continue to show a difference both in the amount of services used and in the source of the services (private physicians as compared with outpatient departments). These differences do not appear to be due to racial differences in the need for medical care among the elderly.

Medicaid was enacted as Title XIX of the Social Security Act in 1965 and provides that the federal government will share with participating states the cost of certain services used by eligible individuals. Currently all states except Arizona participate in Medicaid, as do the District of Columbia, the Virgin Islands, Guam, and Puerto Rico. Federal requirements provide for the mandatory inclusion of groups that are eligible for cash assistance from public

Table 22. USE OF MEDICARE SERVICES BY THE AGED: RATIO OF WHITE TO NONWHITE ENROLLEES BY TYPE OF SERVICE, 1967 and 1976

Type of Reimbursed Services	1967	1976
Hospital Insurance and/or Supplementary Medical Insurance (Total)	1.44	1.13
Hospital Insurance	1.30	1.19
Inpatient Hospital Services	1.36	1.19
Skilled Nursing Facility Services	2.83	1.72
Home Health Agency Services	1.23	0.88
Supplementary Medical Insurance	1.41	1.10
Physician & Other Medical Services	1.49	1.16
Outpatient Services	0.80	0.86
Home Health Agency Services	1.14	0.72

SOURCE: Martin Ruther and Allen Dobson, "Equal Treatment and Unequal Benefits: A Reexamination of the Use of Medicare Services by Race, 1967-1976," Health Care Financing Review 2 (Winter, 1981), pp. 55-83.

programs such as Aid to Families with Dependent Children (AFDC) and Supplemental Security Income (SSI). Eligibility for these programs is determined at the state level using both federally defined, categorical requirements (for example, age, blindness, or disability) and state defined requirements regarding income and resource levels. States also have the option of including within Medicaid "medically needy" persons who meet the categorical but not the financial requirements.[4] Thus, the percentage of poor (by a standard definition) people who are eligible for medical care under Medicaid varies enormously from state to state--from fewer than 20 percent of the poor in many states (particularly in the South) to numbers well in excess of the entire "poor" population in California and New York.

Federal regulations specify a basic set of services that must be provided, and this may vary between the "categorically eligible" and the medically needy. States must provide the categorically eligible with both inpatient and outpatient hospital services; laboratory and X-ray services; skilled nursing facility (SNF) services for individuals 21 and older; family planning services; physician services; and the early and period screening, diagnosis, and treatment (EPSDT) of physical and mental defects in individuals under 21 years of age. In addition, states may opt to cover additional services for categorically eligible persons. States that include the "medically needy" within their Medicaid program may provide either the same set of services provided to the categorically eligible, or services may be restricted to any 7 from an overall list of 16 services. Racial groups may differ in their use of particular services. For example, it appears that a larger proportion of white than black Medicaid recipients are elderly, which has implications for the types of services that the different racial groups are likely to use.

Since states have considerable control over the mix of services that are available to Medicaid recipients, the possibility exists that racial bias affects the mix of services included in a state's Medicaid program. Concern about this aspect of the Medicaid program has risen in North Carolina, where a lawsuit was initiated over proposed Medicaid cutbacks that would have disproportionately affected services used by blacks,[5] and, in Mississippi, where whites constitute 25 percent of the Medicaid population and receive 50 percent of the Medicaid dollars.[6]

Medicaid is the most important source of medical coverage for poor people in the United States. In 1977 there were about 23.8 million recipients at a cost of more than 16 billion dollars.[7] Despite the great importance of the Medicaid program for providing medical care to the least privileged members of society, existing data do not permit even a minimally adequate assessment of the extent of racial/ethnic disparities within the program. Several data problems exist. First, no national data exist on the racial/ethnic characteristics of persons who are eligible to receive services under Medicaid. Thus, it is not possible to develop utilization rates for different groups. Second, many states do not report the race of recipients to the Health Care Financing Administration (HCFA). Thus, in the data published by HCFA, race-specific information is not available for 35 percent of Medicaid recipients and for 28 percent of all Medicaid payments. Third, the racially specific data that are available are only for the two categories, white and "other."

The consequences of these severe data problems are seen in Table 23, which presents data on overall racial distribution of Medicaid recipients and payments. The most striking things about the table are the extent of the missing data, which precludes any conclusions about racial trends, and the absence of any base from which rates of use could be developed.

The available data on the Medicaid program are of very limited usefulness. Table 24 shows the percentage of all Medicaid recipients,

Table 23. PERCENT DISTRIBUTION OF MEDICAID RECIPIENTS AND PAYMENTS, BY RACE, FISCAL YEAR 1977

	White	All Other	Unknown	Total
Recipients	37.0	28.0	35.0	100.0
Payments	50.0	22.0	28.0	100.0

SOURCE: Health Care Financing Administration. Unpublished tables.

Table 24. PERCENTAGE OF ALL MEDICAID RECIPIENTS RECEIVING EACH TYPE OF COVERED SERVICE, FISCAL YEAR, 1977

Service	Total	White	Other Than white
Inpatient Hospital			
General Hospital	15.9	18.2	16.7
Mental Hospital	0.4	0.4	0.1
Skilled Nursing Facility	2.6	3.8	0.8
Intermediate Care Facility			
For Mentally Retarded	0.4	0.7	0.2
All Other	3.1	6.5	1.3
Physician	67.7	71.2	68.8
Dental	19.5	20.1	19.5
Other Practitioners	12.4	13.5	11.8
Outpatient Hospital	36.3	36.1	40.0
Clinic Services	7.0	6.5	10.1
Laboratory and Radiologic	23.1	18.1	17.3
Home Health	1.6	0.7	0.4
Prescribed Drugs	64.7	64.3	62.0
Family Planning	5.6	5.4	6.6
Other Care	13.7	11.8	8.4

SOURCE: Health Care Financing Administration, 1977 State Tables (35, 36, 37), unpublished.

by race, receiving each type of covered service in fiscal year 1977.[8] For most categories, a slightly greater percentage of white enrollees than black enrollees received services. Blacks, however, were slightly more likely than whites to have received clinic and outpatient hospital services. The most striking racial difference, however, was in the use of skilled nursing and intermediate care facilities. The significance of this difference is magnified by the fact that, although relatively few Medicaid recipients receive care in such facilities, more than 40 percent of all expenditures under Medicaid go to skilled nursing and intermediate care facilities.[9] (The topic of race and nursing home use is the subject of Chapter 3 of this report.)

The fact that per-capita Medicaid expenditures are smaller for nonwhites than for whites for most categories raises a question about racial characteristics of those who are eligible for Medicaid and those who receive medical services through the program. The question of whether the racial difference reflects the needs of beneficiaries cannot be answered.

REFERENCES

1. Martin Ruther and Allen Dobson, "Equal Treatment and Unequal Benefits: A Reexamination of the Use of Medicare Services by Race, 1967-1976," Health Care Financing Review 2 (Winter 1981), pp. 55-83.
2. Karen Davis, National Health Insurance, Benefits, Costs and Consequences, (Washington, D.C.: The Brookings Institution, 1975) p. 53.
3. Ruther and Dobson.
4. For a summary of state variations in reimbursement policies and eligibility requirements under Medicaid, see Medicaid/Medicare Management Institute. Data on the Medicaid Program: Eligibility, Services, Expeditions, 1979 Edition (Revised) (Baltimore, MD: Health Care Financing Adminstration, DHEW, 1979).
5. Sylvia Drew Ivie, "Ending Discrimination in Health Care: A Dream Deferred," Presentation before the U.S. Civil Rights Commission, April 15, 1980, p. 37.
6. Aaron Shirley, Presentation before the U.S. Civil Rights Commission on the Federal Role in Rural Health Care Delivery, April 15, 1980.
7. Medicaid/Medicare Management Institute.
8. Health Care Financing Administration, "Medicaid State Tables," 1977, unpublished, 1980.
9. Medicaid/Medicare Management Institute, p. 34.

APPENDIX B

RELEVANT PORTIONS OF THE TITLE VI REGULATIONS

§ 80.3 Discrimination prohibited.

(a) *General.* No person in the United States shall, on the ground of race, color, or national origin be excluded from participation in, be denied the benefits of, or be otherwise subjected to discrimination under any program to which this part applies.

(b) *Specific discriminatory actions prohibited.* (1) A recipient under any program to which this part applies may not, directly or through contractual or other arrangements, on ground of race, color, or national origin:

(i) Deny an individual any service, financial aid, or other benefit provided under the program;

(ii) Provide any service, financial aid, or other benefit to an individual which is different, or is provided in a different manner, from that provided to others under the program;

(iii) Subject an individual to segregation or separate treatment in any matter related to his receipt of any service, financial aid, or other benefit under the program;

(iv) Restrict an individual in any way in the enjoyment of any advantage or privilege enjoyed by others receiving any service, financial aid, or other benefit under the program;

(v) Treat an individual differently from others in determining whether he satisfies any admission, enrollment, quota, eligibility, membership or other requirement or condition which individuals must meet in order to be provided any service, financial aid, or other benefit provided under the program;

(vi) Deny an individual an opportunity to participate in the program through the provision of services or otherwise or afford him an opportunity to do so which is different from that afforded others under the program (including the opportunity to participate in the program as an employee but only to the extent set forth in paragraph (c) of this section).

(vii) Deny a person the opportunity to participate as a member of a planning or advisory body which is an integral part of the program.

(2) A recipient, in determining the types of services, financial aid, or other benefits, or facilities which will be provided under any such program, or the class of individuals to whom, or the situations in which, such services, financial aid, other benefits, or facilities will be provided under any such program, or the class of individuals to be afforded an opportunity to participate in any such program, may not, directly or through contractual or other arrangements, utilize criteria or methods of administration which have the effect of subjecting individuals to discrimination because of their race, color, or national origin, or have the effect of defeating or substantially impairing accomplishment of the objectives of the program as respect individuals of a particular race, color, or national origin.

(3) In determining the site or location of a facilities, an applicant or recipient may not make selections with the effect of excluding individuals from, denying them the benefits of, or subjecting them to discrimination under any programs to which this regulation applies, on the ground of race, color, or national origin; or with the purpose or effect of defeating or substantially impairing the accomplishment of the objectives of the Act or this regulation.

(4) As used in this section, the services, financial aid, or other benefits provided under a program receiving Federal financial assistance shall be deemed to include any service, financial aid, or other benefits provided in or through a facility provided with the aid of Federal financial assistance.

(5) The enumeration of specific forms of prohibited discrimination in this paragraph and paragraph (c) of this section does not limit the generality of the prohibition in paragraph (a) of this section.

(6)(i) In administering a program regarding which the recipient has previously discriminated against persons on the ground of race, color, or national origin, the recipient must take affirmative action to overcome the effects of prior discrimination.

(ii) Even in the absence of such prior discrimination, a recipient in administering a program may take affirmative action to overcome the effects of conditions which resulted in limiting participation by persons of a particular race, color, or national origin.

(c) *Employment practices.* (1) Where a primary objective of the Federal financial assistance to a program to which this regulation applies is to provide employment, a recipient may not (directly or through contractual or other arrangements) subject an individual to discrimination on the ground of race, color, or national origin in its employment practices under such program (including recruitment or recruitment advertising, employment, layoff or termination, upgrading, demotion, or transfer, rates of pay or other forms of compensation, and use of facilities), including programs where a primary objective of the Federal financial assistance is (i) to reduce the employment of such individuals or to help them through employment to meet subsistence needs, (ii) to assist such individuals through employment to meet expenses incident to the commencement or continuation of their education or training, (iii) to provide work experience which contributes to the education or training of such individuals, or (iv) to provide remunerative activity to such individuals who because of handicaps cannot be readily absorbed in the competitive labor market. The following, under existing laws, have one of the above objectives as a primary objective:

(*a*) Projects under the Public Works Acceleration Act, Public Law 87-658, 42 U.S.C. 2641-2643.

(*b*) Work-study under the Vocational Education Act of 1963, as amended, 20 U.S.C. 1371-1374.

(*c*) Programs assisted under laws listed in Appendix A as respects employment opportunities provided thereunder, or in facilities provided thereunder, which are limited, or for which preference is given, to students, fellows, or other persons in training for the same or related employments.

(*d*) Assistance to rehabilitation facilities under the Vocational Rehabilitation Act, 29 U.S.C. 32-34, 41a and 41b.

(2) The requirements applicable to construction employment under any such program shall be those specified in or pursuant to Part III of Executive Order 11246 or any Executive order which supersedes it.

(3) Where a primary objective of the Federal financial assistance is not to provide employment, but discrimination on the ground of race, color, or national origin in the employment practices of the recipient or other persons subject to the regulation tends, on the ground of race, color, or national origin, to exclude individuals from participation in, to deny them the benefits of, or to subject them to discrimination under any program to which this regulation applies, the foregoing provisions of this paragraph (c) shall apply to the employment practices of the recipient or other persons subject to the regulation, to the extent necessary to assure equality of opportunity to, and nondiscriminatory treatment of, beneficiaries.

(d) *Indian Health and Cuban Refugee Services.* An individual shall not be deemed subjected to discrimination by reason of his exclusion from the benefits of a program limited by Federal law to individuals of a particular race, color, or national origin different from his.

(e) *Medical emergencies.* Notwithstanding the foregoing provisions of this section, a recipient of Federal financial assistance shall not be deemed to have failed to comply with paragraph (a) of this section if immediate provision of a service or other benefit to an individual is necessary to prevent his death or serious impairment of his health, and such service or other benefit cannot be provided except by or through a medical institution which refuses or fails to comply with paragraphs (a) of this section.

(Sec. 601, 602, 604, Civil Rights Act of 1964; 78 Stat. 252, 253, 42 U.S.C. 2000d, 2000d-1, 2000d-3) [29 FR 16298, Dec. 4, 1964, as amended at 38 FR 17979, 17982, July 5, 1973]

APPENDIX C

GUIDELINES FOR COMPLIANCE OF NURSING HOMES AND SIMILAR FACILITIES WITH TITLE VI OF THE CIVIL RIGHTS ACT OF 1964

Section 601 of Title VI of the Civil Rights Act of 1964 provides:

> No person in the United States, shall, on the ground of race, color, or national origin, be excluded from participation in, be denied the benefits of, or be subjected to discrimination under any program or activity receiving Federal financial assistance.

Nursing homes or similar facilities[1] that are in compliance with Title VI of the Civil Rights Act are characterized by an absence of separation, discrimination,[2] or other distinction on the basis of race, color, or national origin in any activity conducted by, for, or in the institution affecting the care and treatment of residents.

Compliance with Title VI requires adherence to the following policies and practices:

1. Admission to the Nursing Home:

a. All residents are admitted to the facility without discrimination and no inquiries are made regarding race, color, or national origin prior to admission. The nursing home utilizes its referral sources in a manner which assures an equal opportunity for admission to persons without regard to race, color, or national origin in relation to the population of the service area or potential service area. Where there is a significant variation between the racial or ethnic composition of the resident census and available population census data for the service area or potential service area, the nursing home has a responsibility to determine the reason for such

---

[1]The term "nursing home" as used in this document applies to "extended care facilities, skilled nursing homes and intermediate and domiciliary care homes and similar facilities."

[2]The word "discrimination" as used throughout this document shall be understood to mean "discrimination on account of race, color, or national origin" as used in Section 601, Title VI of the Civil Rights Act of 1964, Public Law 88-352, approved July 2, 1964.

variation and take whatever action may be necessary to correct any discrimination.

b. Admission is not restricted to members of any group or order which discriminates.

c. Nursing home policies regarding deposits, extension of credit and other financial matters are applied uniformly and without regard to race.

d. Information regarding the price and availability of accommodations is uniformly made available to all without regard to race, color, or national origin.

2. Records:

Records are maintained uniformly without discrimination for all residents. Identification by race, color and national origin on records is not considered to be discriminatory and may be used to demonstrate compliance with Title VI.

3. Services and Physical Facilities Provided by the Nursing Home:

a. Residents' privileges and care services such as medical and dental care, nursing, laboratory services, pharmacy, physical, occupational and recreational therapies, social services, volunteer services, dietary service, and housekeeping services are provided on a nondiscriminatory basis.

b. Physical facilities including lounges, dining facilities, lavatories and beauty and barber shops are provided and used without discrimination.

c. Rules of courtesy are uniformly applied without regard to race, color, or national origin in all situations including face-to-face contact and written records and communications.

d. Assignment of staff to residents is not governed by the race, color, or national origin of either resident or staff.

e. Nursing homes which formerly had dual facilities (buildings, waiting rooms, entrances, dining facilities, etc.) have a particular responsibility to demonstrate that such facilities are no longer being operated in a discriminatory manner.

4. Room Assignments and Transfers:

a. Residents are assigned to rooms, wards, floors, sections, buildings, and other areas without regard to race, color, or national origin. Such assignment will result in a degree of multi-racial occupancy of multi-bed accommodations which reflects the proportion of minority use of the facility.

b. Residents are not asked whether they are willing to share accommodations with persons of a different race, color, or national origin. Requests from residents for transfer to other rooms in the same class of accommodations are not honored if based on racial or ethnic considerations. Exceptions may be made only if the attending physician or nursing home administrator certifies in writing that in his judgement there are valid medical reasons or special compelling circumstances in the individual case. However, such certifications may not be used to permit segregation as a routine practice in the facility.

5. Attending Physicians' Privileges:

Privileges of attending residents in the nursing home are granted to physicans and other health professionals without discrimination.

6. Notification of Availability of Services and Nondiscrimination Policy:

a. The nursing home has adopted and where appropriate provided its residents, employees, attending physicians, and others providing services to residents with copies of written statements which set forth the nursing home's nondiscrimination policies and practices. These policies are included in any publication of staff regulations or public information brochures, kept current, and periodically reviewed with employees.

b. The nursing home effectively conveys to the community, to hospitals and other referral sources, its nondiscriminatory policy and the nature and extent of services available.

7. Referrals:

Nursing home referrals, including but not limited to referrals to other facilities and care programs, are made in a manner which does not result in discrimination.

Revised and Issued by:
Office for Civil Rights
Department of Health,
Education, and Welfare

Leon E. Panetta, Director
November 1969

APPENDIX D

HILL-BURTON COMMUNITY SERVICE REGULATIONS

Authority: Sec. 215, 1525, 1602(6), Public Health Service Act as amended; 58 Stat 690, 88 Stat. 2249, 88 Stat. 2259; 42 U.S.C. 216, 300m–4, 300o–1(6).

Subpart G—Community Service

§ 124.601 Applicability.

The provisions of this subpart apply to any recipient of Federal assistance under Title VI or XVI of the Public Health Service Act that has given an assurance that it would make the facility or portion thereof assisted available to all persons residing (and, in the case of Title XVI assisted applicants, employed), in the territorial area it serves. This assurance is referred to in this subpart as the "community service assurance."

§ 124.602 Definitions.

As used in this subpart—

"Act" means the Public Health Service Act, as amended.

"Facility" means the an entity that received assistance under Title VI or Title XVI of the Act and provided a community service assurance.

"Fiscal year" means facility's fiscal year.

"Secretary" means the Secretary of Health, Education, and Welfare or his delegatee.

"Service area" means the geographic area designated as the area served by the facility in the most recent State plan approved by the Secretary under Title VI, except that, at the request of the facility, the Secretary may designate a different area proposed by the facility when he determines that a different area is appropriate based on the criteria in 42 CFR 53.1(d).

"State agency" means the agency of a state fully or conditionally designated by the Secretary as the State health planning and development agency of the State under section 1521 of the Act.

§ 124.603 Provision of services.

(a) *General.*

(1) In order to comply with its community service assurance, a facility shall make the services provided in the facility or portion thereof constructed, modernized, or converted with Federal assistance under Title VI or XVI of the Act available to all persons residing (and, in the case of facilities assisted under Title XVI of the Act, employed) in the facility's service area without discrimination on the ground of race, color, national origin, creed, or any other ground unrelated to an individual's need for the service or the availability of the needed service in the facility. Subject to paragraph (b) (concerning emergency services) a facility may deny services to persons who are unable to pay for them unless those persons are required to be provided uncompensated services under the provisions of Subpart F.

(2) A person is residing in the facility's service area for purposes of this section if the person:

(i) is living in the service area with the intention to remain there permanently or for an indefinite period;

(ii) is living in the service area for purposes of employment; or

(iii) is living with a family member who resides in the service area.

(b) *Emergency services.*

(1) A facility may not deny emergency services to any person who resides (or, in the case of facilities assisted under Title XVI of the Act, is employed) in the facility's service area on the ground that the person is unable to pay for those services.

(2) A facility may discharge a person that has received emergency services, or may transfer the person to another facility able to provide necessary services, when the appropriate medical personnel determine that discharge or transfer will not subject the person to a substantial risk of deterioration in medical condition.

(c) *Third party payor programs.*

(1) The facility shall make arrangements, if eligible to do so, for reimbursement for services with:

(i) Those principal State and local governmental third-party payors that provide reimbursement for services that is not less than the actual costs, as determined in accordance with accepted cost accounting principles; and

(ii) Federal governmental third-party programs, such as medicare and medicaid.

(2) The facility shall take any necessary steps to insure that admission to and services of the facility are available to beneficiaries of the governmental programs specified in subparagraph (1) of this paragraph without discrimination or preference because they are beneficiaries of those programs.

(d) *Exclusionary admissions policies.* A facility is out of compliance with its community service assurance if it uses an admission policy that has the effect of excluding persons on a ground other than those permitted under paragraph (a) of this section. Illustrative applications of this requirement are described in the following paragraphs:

(1) A facility has a policy or practice of admitting only those patients who are referred by physicians with staff privileges at the facility. If this policy or practice has the effect of excluding persons who reside (or for Title XVI facilities, are employed) in the community from the facility because they do not have a private family doctor with staff privileges at the facility, the facility would not be in compliance with its assurance. The facility is not required to abolish its staff physician admissions policy as a usual method for admission. However, to be in compliance with its community service assurance it must make alternative arrangements to assist area residents who would otherwise be unable to gain admission to obtain services available in the facility. Examples of alternative arrangements a facility might use include:

(i) authorizing the individual's physician, if licensed and otherwise qualified, to treat the patient at the facility even though the physician does not have staff privileges at the facility;

(ii) for those patients who have no physician, obtaining the voluntary agreement of physicians with staff privileges at the facility to accept referrals of such patients, perhaps on a rotating basis;

(iii) if an insufficient number of physicians with staff privileges agree to participate in a referral arrangement, requiring acceptance of referrals as a condition to obtaining or renewing staff privileges;

(iv) establishing a hospital-based primary care clinic through which patients needing hospitalization may be admitted; or

(v) hiring or contracting with qualified physicians to treat patients who do not have private physicians.

(2) A facility, as required, is a qualified provider under the Title XIX medicaid program, but few or none of the physicians with staff privileges at the facility or in a particular department or sub-department of the facility will treat medicaid patients. If the effect is that some medicaid patients are excluded from the facility or from any service provided in the facility, the facility is not in compliance with its community service assurance. To be in compliance a facility does not have to require all of its staff physicians to accept medicaid. However, it must take steps to ensure that medicaid beneficiaries have full access to all of its available services. Examples of steps that may be taken include:

(i) obtaining the voluntary agreement of a reasonable number of physicians with staff privileges at the facility and in each department or sub-department to accept referral of medicaid patients, perhaps on a rotating basis;

(ii) if an insufficient number of physicians with staff privileges agree to participate in a referral arrangement, requiring acceptance of referrals as a condition to obtaining or renewing staff privileges;

(iii) establishing a clinic through which medicaid beneficiaries needing hospitalization may be admitted; or

(iv) hiring or contracting with physicians to treat medicaid patients.

(3) A facility requires advance deposits (pre-admission or pre-service deposits) before admitting or serving patients. If the effect of this practice is that some persons are denied admission or service or face substantial delays in gaining admission or service solely because they do not have the necessary cash on hand, this would constitute a violation of the community service assurance. While the facility is not required to forego the use of a deposit policy in all situations, it is required to make alternative arrangements to ensure that persons who probably can pay for the services are not denied them simply because they do not have the available cash at the time services are requested. For example, many employed persons and persons with other collateral do not have savings, but can pay hospital bills on an installment basis, or can pay a small deposit. Such persons may not be excluded from admission or denied services because of their inability to pay a deposit.

§ 124.604 Posted notice.

(a) The facility shall post notices, which the Secretary supplies in English and Spanish, in appropriate areas of the facility, including but not limited to the admissions area, the business office and the emergency room.

(b) If in the service area of the facility the "usual language of households" of ten percent or more of the population, according to the most recent figures published by the Bureau of the Census, is other than English or Spanish, the facility shall translate the notice into that language and post the translated notice on signs substantially similar in size and legibility to, and posted with, those supplied under paragraph (a).

(c) The facility shall make reasonable efforts to communicate the contents of the posted notice to persons who it has reason to believe cannot read the notice.

§ 124.605 Reporting and record maintenance requirements.

(a) *Reporting requirements.*

(1) *Timing of reports.*

(i) A facility shall submit to the Secretary a report to assist the Secretary in determining compliance with this subpart once every three fiscal years, on a schedule to be prescribed by the Secretary. The report required by this section shall be submitted not later than 90 days after the end of the fiscal year, unless a longer period is approved by the Secretary for good cause shown.

(ii) A facility shall also submit the required report whenever the Secretary determines, and so notifies the facility in writing, that a report is needed for proper administration of the program. In this situation the facility shall submit the report specified in this section for the filing of reports, within 90 days after receiving notice from the Secretary, or within 90 days after the close of the fiscal year, whichever is later.

(2) *Content of report.* The report must be submitted on a form prescribed by the Secretary and must include information that the Secretary prescribes to permit a determination of whether a facility has met its obligations under this subpart.

(3) The facility shall provide a copy of any report to the HSA for the area when submitting it to the Secretary.

(4) *Institution of suit.* Not later than 10 days after being served with a summons or complaint, the applicant shall notify the Regional Health Administrator for the Region of HEW in which it is located of any legal action brought against it alleging that it has failed to comply with the requirements of this subpart.[1]

(b) *Record maintenance requirements.*

(1) A facility shall maintain, make available for public inspection consistent with personal privacy, and provide to the Secretary on request, any records necessary to document its compliance requirements of this subpart in any fiscal year, including documents from which information required to be reported under paragraph (a) of this section was obtained. A facility shall maintain these records until 180 days following the close of the Secretary's investigation under § 124.606(a).

§ 124.606 Investigation and enforcement.

(a) *Investigations.*

(1) The Secretary periodically investigates the compliance of facilities with the requirements of this subpart, and investigates complaints.

(2)(i) A complaint is filed with the Secretary on the date on which the following information is received in the Office of the Regional Health Administrator for the Region of HEW in which the facility is located:

(A) The name and address of the person making the complaint or on whose behalf the complaint is made;

(B) The name and location of the facility;

(C) The date or approximate date on which the event complained of occurred, and

(D) A statement of what actions the complainant considers to violate the requirements of this subpart.

(ii) The Secretary promptly provides a copy of the complaint to each facility named in the complaint.

(3) When the Secretary investigates a facility, the facility shall provide to the Secretary on request any documents, records and other information concerning its operations that relate to the requirements of this subpart.

(4) The Act provides that if the Secretary dismisses a complaint or the Attorney General has not brought an action for compliance within six months from the date on which the complaint is filed, the person filing it may bring a private action to effectuate compliance with the assurance. If the Secretary determines that he will be unable to issue a decision on a complaint or otherwise take appropriate action within the six month period, he may, based on priorities for the disposition of complaints that are established to promote the most effective use of enforcement resources, or on the request of the complainant, dismiss the complaint without a finding as to compliance prior to the end of the six month period, but no earlier than 45 days after the complaint is filed.

(b) *Enforcement.*

(1) If the Secretary finds, based on his investigation under paragraph (a) of this section, that a facility did not comply with the requirements of this subpart, he may take any action authorized by law to secure compliance, including but not limited to voluntary agreement or a request to the Attorney General to bring an action against the facility for specific performance.

(2) If the Secretary finds, based on his investigation under paragraph (a) of this section, that a facility has limited the availability of its services in a manner proscribed by this subpart, he may, in addition to any other action that he is authorized to take in accordance with the Act, require the facility to establish an effective affirmative action plan that in his judgment is designed to insure that its services are made available in accordance with the requirements of this subpart.

§ 124.607 Agreements with State agencies.

(a) Where the Secretary finds that it will promote the purposes of this subpart, and the State agency is able and willing to do so, he may enter into an agreement with the State agency for

[1] The addresses of the Regional Office of HEW are set out in 45 C.F.R. 5.31.

the State agency to assist him in administering this subpart in the State.

(b) Under an agreement, the State agency will provide the Secretary with any assistance he requests in any one or more of the following areas, as set out in the agreement:

(1) Investigation of complaints of noncompliance;

(2) Monitoring the compliance of facilities with the requirements of this subpart;

(3) Review of affirmative action plans submitted under § 124.606(b);

(4) Review of reports submitted under § 124.605;

(5) Making initial decisions for the Secretary with respect to compliance, subject to appeal by any party to the Secretary or review by the Secretary on his own initiative; and

(6) Application of any sanctions available to it under State law (such as license revocation or termination of State assistance) against facilities determined to be out of compliance with the requirements of this subpart.

(c) A State agency may use funds received under section 1525 of the Act to pay for expenses incurred in the course of carrying out this agreement.

(d) Nothing in this subpart precludes any State from taking any action authorized by State law regarding the provision of services by any facility in the State as long as the action taken does not prevent the Secretary from enforcing the requirements of this subpart.

Appendix I

SUMMARY OF PUBLIC COMMENTS AND DEPARTMENT'S ACTIONS ON THE UNCOMPENSATED SERVICES AND COMMUNITY SERVICE REGULATIONS

The public comments and the Department's actions on the proposed rules are summarized below. The discussion proceeds sequentially through the regulations. In order to ease understanding of the comments and the Department's response, a brief background statement of the existing and proposed rules precedes each section.

Uncompensated Services

I. Applicability of the rules.

A. Background.

The present rules, set out at 42 CFR 53.111, apply only to Title VI facilities. They apply to facilities assisted with grants for 20 years after completion of construction and to facilities assisted with loans or loan guarantees during the period in which the loan remains unpaid. 42 CFR 53.111(a).

The proposed rules retained the policies of the present rules for Title VI facilities, adding a definition of the term "completion of construction." For Title XVI assisted facilities, the rules applied "at all times" following approval of the Title XVI application, except where the facility assisted did not provide health services when approved. In that case, the rules became applicable when the facility began to provide services. Proposed 42 CFR 124.501.

B. Public comment.

1. Consumers generally opposed the 20 year limit for Title VI facilities as proposed. A large number argued that it should be eliminated entirely, on grounds such as the following: substantial consumer need and hospitals' ability to provide services; the alleged failure of the Department and Title VI State agencies to enforce the obligations in the past; the lack of statutory support for the 20 year limit. Many consumers asserted that prior to 1972, when the 20 year limit was established, the duty to provide uncompensated care was essentially unrecognized and that since 1972 enforcement has been inadequate or inconsistent. Several consumers emphasized that the durational limitation is strictly regulatory. Thus, they argue that facilities which received aid before 1972 did not rely on the limitation. According to consumers, the cases cited in the proposed rules as upholding the 20 year limit merely endorse the Department's authority to apply a limitation but would not bar the removal or alteration by the Department of it.

Other consumers, however, acknowledged that 20 years of actually providing services might be "reasonable", as well as politically more acceptable than restoration of an unlimited duty. They therefore suggested various modifications of the durational limitation. The proposals most commonly made were having the 20 years run from (1) the effective date of the new regulations; (2) the date the facility can document its provision of uncompensated care or the completion of construction, whichever is later; or (3) 1972, when the existing regulations were issued, on the theory that there were no compliance standards (and hence no compliance) before that date. If the 20 year limitation were to run from the effective date of the new regulations, a few comments suggested that the regulations provide for a credit for years in which a facility met the "3%" or "10%" level of care under the present regulations. Consumer comments also urged that if the present 20 year limit is maintained, it be enforced retrospectively.

2. Another consumer suggestion was that the supplemental programs included in the Federal assistance base upon which the 10% compliance level is calculated should be added to § 124.501(a), thereby making these regulations applicable to those supplementary programs.

3. Provider comments consistently supported the proposed retention of the Title VI time limits on the uncompensated services obligation. It was argued that the durational limit is statutorily required, i.e., that the obligation to the government should last only as long as the government's right of recovery (section 609 of the Act) and that the term "reasonable volume" implies an absolute dollar amount of services that is inconsistent with an open-ended obligation. Numerous providers also argued that eliminating or extending the durational limitation now would constitute "impairment of contract", particularly with respect to those facilities assisted after 1972. They argued that any extension of the obligation would impair their long-term financial solvency and divert funds from patient care, and that facilities that have undertaken long-term financial plans and commitments relying on their limited obligations under the present regulations would be significantly harmed.

4. Providers generally opposed the applicability of the uncompensated services assurance without a durational limitation for Title XVI assisted facilities. See proposed § 124.501(b)(2). Some asserted that the perpetual obligation was unauthorized, and that the period of obligation should be the same as for Title VI assisted facilities. Some argued that the Department has misinterpreted the statutory language "at all times," and that the phrase only meant "at all times" during the period in which the obligation applies (that is, 20 years). Providers also expressed the view that it would be prohibitively costly to assume an open-ended obligation and that the net effect of such a rule would be to discourage providers from seeking assistance under Title XVI, a result not intended by Congress. Others argued that the effect of the rule would be to perpetually penalize private-pay patients, who must bear the cost of the uncompensated services provided.

5. A few provider and government comments opposed the clarification of the term "completion of construction" in the proposed rules. They argued that this change would only cause confusion, since for most Title VI facilities the commencement of the obligation is already clearly established.

C. Department's Actions and Response

Although the Department has retained the 20 year period of obligation for Title VI assisted facilities it has made one change that is responsive to those comments that urged that the 20 year period should not be used to "forgive" non-compliance during the 20 year period. Section 124.501(b)(1) now permits lengthening or shortening of the durational limitations for Title VI facilities, to be consistent with the deficit make-up and excess compliance provisions of § 124.503 (b) and (c). The concept underlying those sections is that Title VI facilities undertook to provide a total "volume" of services. The size of that volume is a function of both the annual compliance level and the remaining period of obligation, but it is in essence a fixed amount of services. That being the case, facilities that fail to provide that volume before their 20 year period of obligation expires should not benefit from their failure, while facilities that more than meet their obligation in some years should be credited with the extra amount of services provided. These considerations dictated adjustment of the period of obligation. The discussion below of the compliance level and deficit and excess compliance provisions explains the Department's position more fully.

APPENDIX E

CASE STUDY: COOK v. OCHSNER*

Chapter 5 indicates that the Office for Civil Rights (OCR) in the Department of Health and Human Services (DHHS) is undertaking more rigorous enforcement of its civil rights-related responsibilities in the health care field. It may, therefore, be useful to review the status of the decade-long dispute concerning the discriminatory practices of New Orleans hospitals. It is in the context of this dispute that OCR first exercised a more expansive view of its civil rights authority and demonstrated its ability to assess the compliance of health facilities with civil rights laws. This controversy also brings into focus the problems of applying Title VI to the peculiar circumstances of health care delivery, first for OCR, and subsequently to DHHS's administrative decision-making apparatus and the courts.

The original lawsuit, Cook v. Ochsner Foundation Hospital et al., was filed in 1970 by black residents of metropolitan New Orleans who alleged that New Orleans hospitals were engaged in racial discriminatory practices in violation of Title VI and were not providing a "community service" or "uncompensated services" in violation of their obligations as recipients of Hill-Burton funding. In May 1971, DHEW was added as a party defendant under the allegation that DHEW had failed to provide for an enforcement program under Title VI and Hill-Burton and had allowed the defendant hospitals to operate in violation of their Title VI and Hill-Burton obligations.

By agreement of the parties, the Hill-Burton issues and the Title VI issues were severed and litigated as separate lawsuits. The ensuing litigation of the Hill-Burton issues in Cook resulted in several landmark interpretations of the "uncompensated service" and "community service" obligations of Hill-Burton hospitals and was largely responsible for the issuance of the first federal regulations in 1972 and for the judicially mandated enforcement efforts taken by DHEW since that time.

---

*Prepared as background for the IOM Committee by Kenneth Wing, University of North Carolina School of Law, Chapel Hill, North Carolina.

The Cook litigation had a similar impact on the Title VI enforcement effort. While the Hill-Burton issues were being tried by the courts, the racial discrimination issues were largely ignored. In 1974, however, after plaintiffs exhibited a renewed interest in litigating the discrimination issues, a formal settlement was negotiated between plaintiffs and defendant DHEW under which plaintiffs agreed to dismiss the allegations against DHEW, if DHEW's OCR would undertake compliance reviews of the defendant hospitals under conditions listed in a court-approved timetable.

OCR's attempt to assess the services delivered by the 18 defendant hospitals met with resistance; several of the hospitals initially refused to provide OCR with any compliance data and only did so under court order.

OCR also faced the difficulty of formulating for the first time the form and amount of data that they would require to assess compliance by a hospital with the Title VI assurance and of determining in measurable terms their interpretation of what constituted compliance with Title VI.

Relying heavily on the concepts of compliance that had been developed in reviews of educational institutions, the data request that was finally devised asked primarily for two kinds of data: data on the racial composition and privileges of staff physicians and data on total inpatient and emergency room admissions broken down by race, method of payment, and source of referral. The data request did not ask for a breakdown of services by service area within the facilities, or request a description of the services actually delivered, or in any way try to assess appropriateness or quality of treatment.

But even the available data were difficult to collect. Much was collected by OCR personnel collating information from hospital and patient records. The entire data-collection effort required several years and a major commitment of OCR regional office and central office staff.

In 1977 OCR announced its findings with regard to the New Orleans hospitals under investigation. OCR found that, prior to 1964, New Orleans hospitals were formally and openly segregated. While there were no laws requiring patient segregation, there is little doubt that state and local government would enforce this practice of segregation, and hospitals were required by state laws to segregate restrooms, cafeterias, and water fountains for employees and were required to label blood according to the donor's race.

White patients were referred by their physicians to any hospital in New Orleans except Flint-Goodridge, a private hospital affiliated with Dillard University, generally regarded as the hospital for black patients who could pay for their medical services. Blacks, on the other hand, were admitted to either Charity Hospital, the segregated public hospital for indigents of all races, or Flint-Goodridge.

This segregated pattern was perpetuated by the practice of dual admissions. Many physicians maintained staff privileges at two or more hospitals, at least one white and one black, and would admit only white patients to the white hospital and black patients to Charity or Flint-Goodridge.

This pattern of open and governmentally sanctioned segregation was finally broken in 1966. Following the enactment of Medicaid and Medicare, hospitals were required by Title VI to execute non-discrimination assurances as a condition to participation and to terminate discriminatory policies and practices. By 1970 all of the New Orleans hospitals had executed assurances and terminated overt policies of discrimination. Most all-white New Orleans hospitals began admitting black patients as early as 1966.

Nonetheless, OCR's 1974-77 analysis of admission practices by each hospital showed that de facto discrimination still persisted, and hospital care in New Orleans, for all practical purposes, continued to be racially segregated. Of the 16 hospitals in the metropolitan New Orleans area, 75 percent of the black population went to Flint-Goodridge and Charity hospitals. The patient populations of many of the remaining hospitals were virtually all white, and blacks were grossly underrepresented in all hospitals except Flint-Goodridge and Charity.

In general, OCR concluded that the all-white or all-black images of New Orleans hospitals were unchanged since 1966. Many practices that affected hospital service to minorities had continued. For example, the policy and image of Charity Hospital as the "hospital for the poor," allowed most physicians to restrict the number of Medicaid and Medicare patients that they accepted and, consequently, that were admitted to private hospitals. Black physicians were also discouraged from applying for privileges at the predominantly white hospitals by a requirement that applicants for medical staff privileges be members of the local AMA-affiliate medical society, which had traditionally been all white.

Prior to 1964 the medical staff of Flint-Goodridge was predominantly white. After the passage of the Civil Rights Act, the hospital board of trustees enacted a policy prohibiting white physicians from admitting only black patients to the hospital; following the enactment of this policy and the initial assessment of Title VI compliance incident to initial Medicare certification, most of the white physicians dropped their Flint-Goodridge privileges. As of 1978 there was only one white physician practicing at Flint-Goodridge; most of the white physicians who dropped their privileges also stopped treating black patients.

The findings with respect to Hotel Dieu, Mercy, and Southern Baptist hospitals (the hospitals that eventually were found to be out of compliance with Title VI) reflect this segregated pattern of delivery in New Orleans following 1964.

In 1978 the New Orleans population was estimated to be 55 percent black, and the New Orleans standard metropolitan area 33 percent black. Of the patients that Hotel Dieu served, 78.6 percent were from the New Orleans area. Assuming that blacks and whites were served according to their proportion of the population, Hotel Dieu should have served, at the very least, 25.9 percent black patients (78.6 percent of 33 percent). (This assumes that the remaining 21.4 percent of the patients came from totally white populations.) However, Hotel Dieu was only serving 18.4 percent black patients in 1978. This proportion had, however, increased from the 0.2 percent proportion of black patients it served in 1965.

Data on black admissions at Mercy Hospital, Hotel Dieu, and Southern Baptist Hospital are presented in Table 25. Of Mercy Hospital's patients, 89.4 percent were from the New Orleans area. Theoretically, Mercy Hospital should have served, at the very least, 29.5 percent black patients (89.4 percent of 33 percent). However, Mercy Hospital only served 9.2 percent blacks in 1978, an increase from the 0.01 percent black patient population in 1967.

Only 53.3 percent of Southern Baptist's patients were from the New Orleans area. Thus, at the very least, 17.6 percent (53.3 percent of 33 percent) of Southern Baptist's patients should have been black. Yet, in 1978, only 7.4 percent of the patients admitted into Southern Baptist hospital were black. This represented an increase from the 2.8 percent black patients served in 1974. A similar analysis is shown in Table 26, in which method of payment is controlled and shows, again, that race was a factor in admissions to the three hospitals.

Similar patterns were found in the racial composition of the medical staff. At the time of the hearing, there were 55-60 licensed black physicians in the New Orleans area, approximately 2 percent of all the physicians. In 1978, Hotel Dieu had 10 black physicians on its staff, which amounted to 3.0 percent of its medical staff. Mercy Hospital had only two black staff physicians, equaling 0.8 percent of its medical staff, and Southern Baptist had two black staff physicians, or 0.4 percent of its medical staff.

With the exception of one black representative on the lay advisory board of Mercy Hospital, there have been no known black representatives on any of the hospitals' boards of trustees or lay advisory boards.

On July 19, 1977, DHEW notified these three hospitals that it had finished its investigation and that each hospital had been found to be out of compliance with Title VI.

As required by the Title VI regulations, DHEW's OCR and the three hospitals entered into negotiations in an attempt to secure voluntary compliance. These negotiations were protracted and not always amicable. Each of the hospitals denied any discrimination on their part but, nonetheless, agreed to a limited amount of negotiations.

Again, DHEW was faced with a task it had not attempted before--formulating remedial steps for non-complying health facilities. Eventually DHEW made similar requests to all three hospitals. The requests included (1) establish an outpatient primary care clinic where patients needing hospital services would be advanced into the hospital, (2) develop a referral system from outside clinics whereby patients who needed to be admitted would be referred to a staff physician who would take responsibility for admittance and treatment, (3) require as a condition of staff privileges that physicians treat Medicaid patients, (4) find out which physicians provided care for the black community and encourage them to apply for staff privileges, (5) embark on an extensive publicity campaign to change their images in the community as all-white institutions, and (6) appoint leaders of the black community to the hospital's board of trustees and other lay boards.

Table 25. BLACK ADMISSIONS AT THREE NEW ORLEANS HOSPITALS: 1965-78

Mercy Hospital

Year	Total Number Patients	Total Number Black Patients	Percent Black Patients
1967	11,059	77	0.7
1963	11,226	118	1.0
1969	10,368	214	2.1
1971	10,116	433	4.3
1974	9,877	641	6.5
1975	7,991	506	6.0
1977	7,618	716	9.3
1978	7,645	704	9.2

Hotel Dieu Hospital

Year	Total Number Patients	Total Number Black Patients	Percent Black Patients
1965	12,322	19	0.2
1966	11,754	5	0.04
1967	9,559	190	2.0
1968	9,289	217	2.3
1969	8,420	225	2.7
1974	8,779	711	8.1
1975	10,673	1,185	11.1
1976	10,861	1,360	12.5
1977 (8 mo's)	7,867	1,004	13.6
1978	10,660	1,965	18.4

Southern Baptist Hospital

Year	Total Number Patients	Total Number Black Patients	Percent Black Patients
1968		2	
1969		25	
1970		90	
1974	20,591	571	2.8
1975	20,673	729	3.5
1976	20,229	955	4.2
1977	20,680	1,206	5.8
1978	20,731	1,534	7.4

Note: Included are data collected in 1978 while the negotiations and subsequent hearings were taking place.

Table 26. EXPECTED AND ACTUAL BLACK ADMISSIONS, BY SOURCE OF PAYMENT, AT THREE NEW ORLEANS HOSPITALS, 1974

Hotel Dieu Hospital

Method of Payment	Expected Black Patients	Observed Black Patients	Number of Standard Deviations
Private Health Insurance	651	366	11.6
Medicare	334	98	13.5
Medicaid	84	38	5.0
Private Pay	175	46	9.8

Mercy Hospital

Method of Payment	Expected Black Patients	Observed Black Patients	Number of Standard Deviations
Private Health Insurance	728	364	14.1
Medicare	369	75	16.1
Private Pay	236	68	11.3

Southern Baptist Hospital

Method of Payment	Expected Black Patients	Observed Black Patients	Number of Standard Deviations
Private Health Insurance	1229	229	30.7
Medicare	544	49	22.9
Medicaid	51	4	6.6
Private Pay	800	69	26.8
Free Care	157	17	11.3

Hotel Dieu eventually refused to undergo any type of compliance negotiations or submit a corrective action plan to OCR, arguing that it was in compliance with Title VI and could not be required to take any remedial steps.

Mercy Hospital, while denying non-compliance with Title VI, did enter into negotiations and offered to (1) have formal and informal discussions with its medical staff to encourage the staff to admit their black Medicare and Medicaid patients into Mercy Hospital; (2) encourage black physicians in the community to apply for staff privileges; (3) establish a referral system with the New Orleans

Health Corporation Clinics (NOHC), whereby Medicare and/or Medicaid patients in need of inpatient hospital care would be referred to the hospital; and (4) encourage nomination for appointments of blacks to the board of trustees. (Mercy Hospital did not agree to require its staff physicians to treat referral patients; rather it agreed to encourage such referral agreements.)

Southern Baptist Hospital also denied violation of Title VI but agreed to negotiations and eventually to take the following measures: (1) send a letter of inquiry to all hospital staff physicians asking them if they would accept referrals from community health clinics; (2) send a letter to the medical staff reminding them of the hospital's policy of non-discrimination and encouraging them to refer their black patients to the hospital; (3) informally encourage black physicians to apply for staff privileges; (4) pass a resolution reaffirming its policy of non-discrimination in patient referrals; (5) publicize the hospital's policy of non-discrimination; (6) recommend qualified blacks to the board of trustees and make efforts to increase the number of blacks on local advisory boards; and (7) encourage, but not require, staff physicians to treat Medicaid patients. Southern Baptist was operating a clinic at the time of the hearing, but it only admitted the indigent patients of staff physicians. The hospital refused to expand this clinic to include all indigent walk-in patients because the costs would be excessive.

On May 24, 1978, OCR staff determined that further negotiations with the respondent hospitals would be futile; according to required procedures, the cases were referred to the General Counsel of DHEW for enforcement and fund termination proceedings.

The process for terminating funding under Title VI is long and cumbersome--so cumbersome as to discourage DHEW from initiating proceeding in any but the most extreme cases. The initial "trial" of the issue takes place before an administrative law judge (ALJ). The findings of the ALJ can be appealed to the Reviewing Authority, a three-person board appointed by the Secretary that acts as an appellant body. Final decision within the agency is made by the Secretary. This decision is subject to review by the courts. The initial ALJ decision, particularly with regard to fact-finding, has a great deal of importance, but represents only an initial adjudication of the facts and the resulting issues.

The ALJ held hearings from April to June 1979. Many substantive, jurisdictional, and procedural issues were raised by all parties (including representatives of the plaintiffs in the original lawsuit).

The relevant substantive issue can be summarized as two basic questions: (1) do the disparities between treatment of whites and treatment of minorities constitute either present discrimination or vestiges of prior discrimination and (2) if so, what remedies can be required of defendant hospitals?

While exhibiting considerable sympathy for defendants' argument that they were only part of a larger system over which they had little control, the ALJ found that vestiges of prior discrimination continued to exist and that it was unlikely that "time alone" would remedy the situation or prevent discriminatory practices by any of the defendant facilities.

Recognizing that Title VI regulations require remedial steps to eliminate vestiges of prior discrimination, the ALJ then reviewed the substance and history of negotiations between the defendants and OCR and evaluated OCR's proposals. The ALJ felt that reference to a "white-only" image was only the subjective impression argued by the government. Thus it was "not appropriate to eliminate the white-only image, but it is appropriate to inform the public, including the black minority, that the respondent hospitals will comply with the Act and will treat patients without regard to race or color."

The ALJ also downplayed the significance of efforts to recruit black physicians as a remedial requirement, relying heavily on the fact that there are few black physicians in the area. Since there are so few black physicians in New Orleans, the ALJ concluded that no statistical determination of "racial identifiability" of the medical staffs could be made. Therefore nothing over and above the informal recruitment of black physicians (already undertaken by the hospitals) was required.

On the other hand, the ALJ found that the referral agreement between NOHC and the defendant hospitals was a reasonable step to eliminate vestiges of past discrimination. However, these referral agreements did not bind the hospitals' staff physicians to treat these patients. Admittance into the hospitals was still contingent on the decision of a staff physician. The staff physicians were encouraged, but not required, to take referred patients.

The ALJ also found that a requirement to take Medicaid patients as a condition of staff privileges was inappropriate, relying on the facts that no showing had been made that the defendants' medical staffs had engaged in discrimination in patient care or referral and that the physicians were not parties to the proceedings. "While enforcement of equal opportunity requirements on subcontractors may be appropriate, their imposition on subcontractors is only appropriate after they are given the same right to a hearing as in the case of a prime recipient."

The requirement that the respondent set up outpatient clinics was also rejected by the ALJ because the costs were considered excessive.

Finally, the ALJ concluded that qualified blacks must be given serious consideration for membership on the defendants' boards of trustees and advisory boards. The ALJ would not accept an absolute requirement that a certain number of blacks be put on these boards. This conclusion was reached, "because of the remoteness from direct patient contact, and, in the case of Hotel Dieu and Mercy, the requirement of religious order membership for qualification."

Based on these general conclusions regarding DHEW's compliance requests, the ALJ looked at each of the respondents to determine if they were out of compliance with Title VI. He found that, given the racial composition of its patient population, Hotel Dieu was no longer "racially identifiable." However, the hospital was required to take appropriate steps in order to increase utilization by blacks. These requirements included: (1) notify its staff and the public that it would admit and treat patients regardless of race or color, (2) either establish a patient referral system at its existing walk-in clinic or set up a referral agreement with NOHC, and (3) give serious consideration for qualified blacks for boards other than the board of trustees where all members were part of the sponsoring religious order.

Mercy Hospital was found to be "racially identifiable" by patient population. The hospital was required to take appropriate steps in order to reach compliance with Title VI. These requirements included: (1) notify its staff and the public that it would admit and treat patients regardless of race or color, (2) continue its informal efforts to recruit black physicians to its medical staff, and (3) give serious consideration to blacks for board positions. (By the time of the hearing, Mercy Hospital had completed an agreement with NOHC under which Mercy agreed to accept all referrals from the clinic.)

The ALJ found Southern Baptist was also "racially identifiable." However, the ALJ accepted Southern Baptist's compliance proposals as complete and sufficient to eliminate the continuing vestiges of past discrimination and therefore required no specific remedial steps by Southern Baptist.

At this point in the proceeding, many at the OCR view the ALJ decision as little more than a hollow victory. If the factual findings and legal conclusions of the ALJ are upheld through the appellate procedures, the jurisdiction of OCR under Title VI will be severely limited in several ways.

First, the ALJ adopted a limited interpretation of the scope of Title VI. There was little question but that the New Orleans hospitals had practiced racial discrimination in the past and that there continued to be disparities in the services provided to whites and minorities. The ALJ found that there was sufficient linkage between the disparate treatment and the prior discrimination to constitute a violation of Title VI. But in doing so, the ALJ expressed considerable sympathy for the argument that this linkage was complicated by a number of variables beyond the hospitals' control. He also used a 20 percent variance as a criteria in evaluating the materiality of the apparent disparities. Under a slightly different set of circumstances, such a method of analysis would lead to the conclusion that Title VI had not been violated. In particular, it seems evident that this ALJ would not have found discrimination had there not been a clear pattern of discrimination prior to 1966; that is, the ALJ would require a finding of either past or present discriminatory intent in addition to substantial disparities.

Thus, the ALJ's decision calls into question DHEW's (and presumably the DHHS) interpretation of Title VI and the guidelines issued in 1969. A test of discrimination relying so heavily on an overt showing of intent and on such a narrow test of material disparity would limit DHHS' jurisdiction to only the most blatantly discriminatory health facilities.

The ALJ's view of appropriate remedies, even when Title VI has been violated, also follows a conservative pattern. The ALJ rejected virtually all concrete (and controversial) steps proposed by OCR and required little more than expressions of good faith and non-discriminatory intentions by the facilities--again, rejecting the implications of the Title VI regulations and guidelines.

The characterization by the ALJ of the relationship between hospitals and their medical staffs as being primarily contractual also demonstrates the ALJ's view of the limits of OCR's authority in this case.

> This case is concerned with the medical staff relationship. At the origin of the hospital, the hospital management establishes the original medical staff by-laws. These medical staff by-laws provide for procedures or admissions to practice, hospital rules affecting physician procedures, hospital policies, and disciplinary or removal procedures. Once the medical staff by-laws are in place and the hospital is functioning, changes in the by-laws are customarily a subject of negotiation between hospital management and the medical staff represented by a by-law committee. <u>Ultimately, the hospital retains the authority to unilaterally change medical staff by-laws</u>. The hospital's readily apparent need for support and participation by a highly qualified medical staff of physicians acts to restrain the hospital's arbitrary unilateral changes in the by-laws. . . . Upon acceptance [of staff-privileges by a physician] the physicians agree to abide by the by-laws. This arrangement becomes an agreement or contract between the physician and the hospital. The hospital agrees to provide hospital services to patients admitted by the physician. During its term, the contract is subject to change only under its terms. (emphasis added)

OCR has historically taken the position that private physicians, who are participating providers under Medicare, are not covered by Title VI, apparently on the theory that there is no contractual agreement between DHEW/DHHS and individual physicians participating in Medicare--a position that has no apparent basis in law. But paired with the ALJ's narrow view of the incidental obligations of a medical staff physician, this interpretation would virtually quash any effort to enforce Title VI in health facilities unless facilities make discrimination a matter of institutional policy.

It must be noted that the interpretation of the ALJ does not conform to the interpretation of virtually all modern courts of the hospital-physician relationship, at least in the context of medical staff privilege decisions, malpractice liability, or even the Hill-Burton "charity care" obligations.

As indicated earlier, the New Orleans litigation may well be the context within which these (and many other) issues will be adjudicated for the first time. It is possible that all or some of the defendants will negotiate an acceptable settlement and the findings, both favorable and unfavorable to DHHS, will never be tested in the courts. But since it represents the major hospital compliance effort of OCR, the precedential value of whatever outcome is achieved, either through litigation or negotiations, will not be lost on any of the parties to the 10-year dispute or on the provider community.

It also serves as a model, for better or worse, of OCR's technical and administrative capabilities. The manner in which OCR formulated and conducted its data-collection effort and developed the remedial practices that become the focus of the negotiations demonstrate the administrative "state of the art" as OCR enters this "new era" of civil rights enforcement.

APPENDIX F

Speakers Presenting Testimony at the Open Meeting of the Committee on Health Care of Racial/Ethnic Minorities and Handicapped Persons

National Academy of Sciences
June 6, 1980

Mr. Hal Bleakley, American Federation of the Blind

Ms. Susan Conner, National Citizens Coalation for Nursing Home Reform

Ms. Clair Feinson, Consumer Coalition for Health

John L. S. Holloman, Jr., M.D.

Mr. Sanford A. Newman, Center for Law and Social Policy

Mark Ozer, M.D., Mainstream, Inc.

Ms. Sarah Rosenbaum, Children's Defense Fund

Gretchen Schafft, Ph.D., Foundation of the American College of Nursing Home Administrators, Inc.

Mr. Sean Walsh, National Association of Community Health Centers

Ms. Judith Waxman, National Health Law Program